Jeanne Rose's
Kitchen
Cosmetics

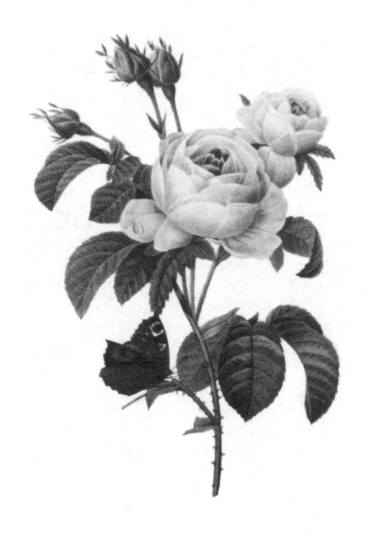

To WONDER WOMAN and her mother
Queen Hippolyte
. . . Wise as Athena and as lovely as Aphrodite
Stronger than Hercules and swifter than Mercury . . . .

Jeanne Rose's
Kitchen
Cosmetics

Using herbs, fruit, & flowers for natural bodycare

Botanical drawings by
Annetta Günter

Herbal Studies Course/Jeanne Rose
San Francisco, California

North Atlantic Books
Berkeley, California

Kitchen Cosmetics

ISBN 1–55643–101–5

Publishers' addresses:

Herbal Studies Course/Jeanne Rose
219 Carl Street
San Francisco, California 94117

North Atlantic Books
2800 Woolsey Street
Berkeley, California 94705

Old herbal prints and photographs
from the author's collection

Cover photo and design by Paula Morrison

Printed in the United States of America

Kitchen Cosmetics is sponsored by the Society for the Study of Native Arts and Sciences, a nonprofit educational corporation whose goals are to develop an ecological and cross-cultural perspective linking various scientific, social and artistic fields; to nurture a holistic view of arts, sciences, humanities, and healing; and to publish and distribute literature on the relationship of mind, body, and nature.

Library of Congress Cataloging in Publication Data:

Rose, Jeanne, 1940—
  Kitchen Cosmetics.

  Bibliography: p. 123
  Includes index.

  1. Cosmetics. I. Title.
TP983.R533 668'.5 77–17077

EDITOR'S NOTE:

All plants, like all medicines, may be dangerous if used improperly—if they are taken internally when prescribed for external use, if they are taken in excess, or if they are taken for too long a time. Allergic reactions and unpredictable sensitivities, particularly to douches, may develop. One way to determine whether you are allergic to any of the recipes contained in this book would be to test the preparations on a small patch of skin before using it on larger portions of the body. Be sure your herbs are fresh and keep conditions of use as sterile as possible.

We do not advocate, endorse, or guarantee the curative effects of any of the substances listed in this book. We have made every effort to see that any botanical that is dangerous or potentially dangerous has been noted as such. When you use herbs, recognize their potency and use them with care.

Epithet

Though sin and Satan hath plunged mankind into an ocean of infirmities, yet the mercy of God which is over all His works maketh grass to grow upon the mountains and herbs for the use of man and hath not only stamped upon them (as upon every man) a distinct form, but also given them particular signatures, whereby a man may read even in legible characters the use of them.

—William Cole
Art of Simpling

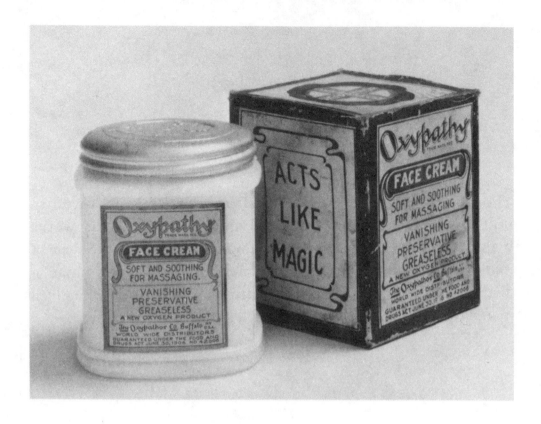

Cosmetics have been with us since men and women first became interested in their appearance. In earlier days some preparations were advertised simply on the basis of what they didn't contain, such as those with No Poisonous Ingredients. Now, with some cosmetics having a price tag higher than an ounce of gold, what is really being sold is hope, such as the cosmetic pictured which "acts like magic." On the other side of the package is the admonition that "Life Is A Constant Struggle Against Oxygen Deficiency," a quote attributed to Pawlow. It makes more sense to me to forget hope and make one's own cosmetics from known, easily available and pure ingredients instead of buying high-priced junk with incomprehensible ingredients from your local drug and department stores.

Preface
Some Rambling Thoughts on Herbal Body Care

IF YOU WANT a natural and wholesome look to your skin, you of course want to use natural and wholesome ingredients, not only on it but *in* it (in yourself of course). The word cosmetic, from the Greek root *Kosmetiko*, really means the *art* of beautifying the body. This art can involve external applications to cover up blemishes and enhance otherwise nondescript features, *or* it can involve techniques for real and permanent beauty. So, you can make quick but temporary changes or gradual and long-lasting ones. Using natural ingredients often found in the kitchen will work in this latter way. The recipes in this book will act upon your body to change it slowly and thus you will become, in time, more attractive, your skin will become more healthy and of course with health comes glowing beauty.

The older meaning of *Kosmea* is to harmonize. This is what we want to do with the herbs and ingredients discussed in the following pages: to harmonize or bring into balance and to normalize skin function. Thus, we shy away from words such as dry or oily skin because this only means that the skin is out of balance, and what we want is to create a balance within the skin and its metabolic function.

The plants in my recipes are chosen for their special relationship to the skin's activity. The effectiveness of these plant preparations depends on the herbal extracts, essential oils and aromatic substances as well as the organic ingredients contained therein. Beautiful skin depends not only on the outer applications but also on the inner application of the plants. So you will also find a few recipes for teas that you should drink regularly. And your inner attitude is important also. Who will say that a person is beautiful if their features are attractive but their visage is dour and unpleasant. Your inner attitude depends on proper nutrition, good and abundant exercise, fresh clean air, sun and adequate sleep.

In the brochure that comes with Dr. R. Hauschka's herbal cosmetics, you will find a statement that exactly concurs with my feelings on herbal preparations:

> ... The unusual quality of these cosmetic preparations was made possible through a combination of complimentary herbal substances which as a totality stimulate the activity of forces necessary to produce a harmonizing effect, though a specific type of skin or a specific dermal condition may demand a particular herbal ingredient. The skin, as it were, will be able to extract and utilize the particular component itself from the cosmetic combination of herbal substances.*

There are, of course, dozens and dozens of recipes and formulations for cosmetics and other body care products that use natural ingredients. Here we will stick to some of the simpler ones. These are the recipes that I use personally on myself and my family, and I have devised them to keep us looking and feeling healthy and attractive. The ingredients are those you would find in your kitchen, and the recipes are my favorite ones for balancing the skin in a totally pure and natural way. I hope that they work for you as well as they have for us.

Enjoy yourself!
Jeanne Rose

*See the Where to Buy It guide on page 118 for a mailing address to receive Dr. Hauschka's brochure.

Contents

Table of Recipes

I

GENERAL HINTS ON USING PLANTS IN COSMETICS

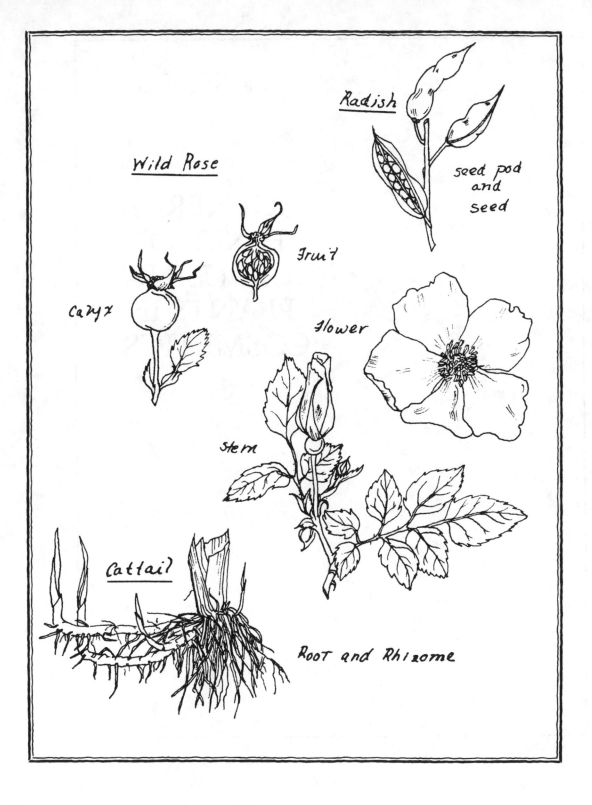

Radish

seed pod
and
seed

Wild Rose

Fruit

Calyx

Flower

Stem

Cattail

Root and Rhizome

An Invitation from the Author

COME OUTSIDE with me into my little garden and see the green things growing there. My garden is bordered by the walls of apartment buildings and the sun can only visit occasionally. It is a green garden with plants planted for fragrance rather than the color of flowers. The main color, green, is the "Colour of Nature," of harmony and balance, a color that has a soothing influence on a disquieted Spirit. As you walk down the brick path, geraniums brush your hand and clothes. They leave the scent of Roses in the air but Rose scent with a cleanly sharp and biting difference. You wonder where the scent is coming from since the little pinkish flowers seem so insignificant. Tweak a leaf and bruise it gently between your fingers. Each of the plants has a unique scent. There are the Rose Geranium, the Nutmeg Geranium, the fresh green apple smell of the Apple Geranium, the Lemon and the Lime Geranium, attar of Rose Geranium, the Lemon-scented Geranium with small curled leaves, the strongly scented Peppermint Geranium with large very fuzzy pale green leaves, spice-scented Lady Mary, the strongly scented Oak-leaved Geranium, as well as Lemony Lemon Verbena, Lemon Balm, Yarrow, Violet, Nasturtium, Dill, Fennel, and the Costmary that smells like Doublemint gum.

My garden also has several types of Roses, traditional Roses, old-timey Roses with their blossoms of old-fashioned scent: there is the Musk Rose, the Eglantine Rose with its fresh green apple smell, *Rosa Gallica*—the Apothecary Rose, the fragrant Damask Rose of long ago, and several striped varieties.

A walk through my garden takes five brief minutes or several long days. But it is mainly a garden of easy care. There are no fancy knot patterns here, but plain herbs, simply laid out and simply cared for. It is first and foremost a garden to be enjoyed and richly savoured. The herbs are all simple to grow and easily used in my kitchen cosmetics.

So walk among the plants, pick some that please you, simmer them in water, and enjoy yourself and the wonderful, beautifying unguents that you will make.

How To Gather Fresh Plants for Processing Into Cosmetics

Herbs ARE ANY PLANTS, their seeds, roots, leafy parts or flowers. Each part should be picked properly to preserve the essence of the plant.

The **herb or leafy part** (as opposed to the root) should be picked in the morning at about 9 A.M. before the sun is very high or very hot and has evaporated all the essential oil of the leaf. Pick only after the dew has dried on the plants. Here in San Francisco this often does not occur until later in the afternoon.

Annuals, those plants that have to be replanted every year, such as Marigolds, can be cut halfway down to the root, tied into small bundles, and hung upside down in a very dry, dark and warm space with circulating air. For example, think of what an attic or a barn would be like and use a space like that. I used to live in a third-floor apartment that had a warm, dry space in the eaves behind the kitchen stove. It worked just fine for drying plants. I also don't necessarily cut down the entire annual but will often cut only a small bunch of the plant at any given time. This way the plant may renew itself once or twice before the growing season is over. Annuals often thrive by having just their leaves picked, without the coarse and longer-to-dry stem.

Perennials and biennials, such as Sage and Thyme, need only have the top third of the plant cut and tied in small bundles to hang. I often pick thick-leaved, scented Geraniums and lay them on fiberglass screens in front of a 250° oven for thirty minutes or so. They have such thick leaves that this quickly drives out some of the moisture so that they dry with more of the color left in.

When hanging the plants, check them daily to see that they are drying and not molding. If there is mold, throw away the affected plants. Make sure air is circulating among all parts of the plant so that they dry evenly and completely.

The **seeds** of plants such as Dill, Fennel, and Caraway are picked when they are ripe (usually they look brown and shrivelled and are intensely fragrant), but before they have fallen to the ground. When the seed pod develops you can tie paper or cheesecloth bags over the heads and let the seeds ripen inside the bags. The seeds will fall into these bags and are then easily removed, packaged, and labelled. The seed pods may also ripen on the plant and then be cut off and placed in brown paper bags to finish ripening and curing. I often use this method, always labelling my paper bags, and then I put the bags on or near the hot water heater to completely dry the seeds.

Roots, such as Comfrey root, are dried by pulling the entire plant out of the ground at the end of the growing season. The roots are washed, broken into smaller pieces and laid on screens to dry. The roots should not touch, and the screens should be put in a dry place. Turn the roots occasionally so that they dry evenly.

Barks are usually peeled in vertical strips from the tree limbs in the fall before the tree goes dormant or in the spring before the juices have come up again. The bark strips can be hung on a clothesline in the sun or in the eaves of your house to dry.

Flowers should be picked daily as they open, after the dew has dried, but before the sun is hot. Pick just below the calyx (see illustration p. 12) and lay them on cheesecloth or screens until they are completely dry.

Simple Methods for Drying Plants

THERE ARE SEVERAL methods for drying plants which I call the Screen Method, the Bunch Method, the Lazy Person Newspaper Way, the Paper Bag Method and the Hanging Cheesecloth Method.

1. For the **Screen Method** use fiberglass screens. Sears stores sell them for windows at a reasonable price, but I prefer the ones my husband makes with fiberglass window screening from the hardware store stapled around wooden frames of 1″ × 1″ lumber. This means you can lay the herb parts *in* the frame and stack the frames one above the other and the herbs will not touch each other. Remember to check the herbs daily; move them around and keep them in a dark, dry and warm place with circulating air.

2. In the **Bunch Method** you tie small bunches of herbs with string and hang them upside down wherever it is dry and there is circulating air.

3. For **Lazy Persons,** take sheets of newspaper and wrap up one or two stalks of semidried herbs. Then hang your newspaper-wrapped herbs in your usual dry, dark and warm place.

4. The **Paper Bag Method** is generally used for seeds and barks. You simply place seed heads or pieces of bark in paper bags and hang them up for further drying.

5. The **Hanging Cheesecloth Method** is best for flowers and herbs. Unwrap long sheets of cheesecloth, which usually come in packages one foot wide and twelve feet long. Thumbtack or staple the cheesecloth across a room one foot below the ceiling. Then pick your plants or flowers and lay them on the cloth where they will dry nicely.

One very important thing to remember is that *you must label* your drying herbs, because once dried they are often difficult to tell apart.

Simple Directions for Making
Creams, Lotions, Ointments Salves, Unguents, Teas, Infusions, Tisanes, and Decoctions

In these directions *always* use an enamel or nonmetal pot.

TEA: For one cup of tea, to drink or as a face wash, bring 10 oz. of water to a rolling boil, prewarm the teapot, add 1 tablespoon of dried herbs (or less) or a largish pinch of fresh herbs and pour the boiling water over them. If you like, add some Honey. Cover the pot and steep to taste, usually 3-5 minutes. Now strain the tea into a cup and drink. Remember that the more herbs you use the stronger the tea will taste. If you use more herbs and steep them longer you will get a more medicinal drink called an infusion.

INFUSION: Prewarm a teapot, add 1 quart of boiling water and throw in a large handful of fresh herbs or an ounce or more of dried herbs. Add some Honey, if desired. Infuse for 10-20 minutes to fully extract all the qualities of the herbs. Strain and drink.

TISANE: A nourishing decoction with some medicinal qualities originally made from barley. This term is now used for a beverage tea made from flowers and is also defined as an infusion of herbs. Use the same directions as for a tea.

DECOCTION: An infusion is steeped while a decoction is boiled. It is usually made from the tougher parts of the plant, the roots, bark or seeds. Put 1 oz. or more herb parts and 1 quart water into a pot. Cover the pot, bring to a boil, and *simmer* for 10-20 minutes or longer. Steep and strain the mixture. Drink it or apply externally.

OINTMENT, CREAM, SALVE: A cosmetic ointment is simply an herb crisped in a solid fat, strained, beaten until cold, and stored away for use. A simple ointment is made with only one herb, a compound is made with two or more herbs.

CERATE, UNGUENT: An ointment is usually made with a solid fat while a cerate is made with a liquid fat and then solidified with wax.

Simmer in a water bath or top of a double boiler 1 oz. of finely crushed or chopped herbs, 8 oz. of oil, plus 1 oz. of white wine. Simmer all together until the wine is boiled off. Cool the mixture a bit, strain out the herbs, add 1 oz. of melted wax, mix together and then beat until cold with a wooden spoon.

MELLITE: A decoction or an infusion made with honey that you use cosmetically is called a mellite. Mix together and simmer 1 oz. of herbs and 10 oz. of water gently for 10-20 minutes. Strain out the herbs, add to the herbal decoction an equal quantity of honey and simmer again until the water has been reduced by half. Another way to make a mellite is to simmer 1 oz. of herbs directly into 10 oz. of honey in a *bain marie* (water bath) for 10-20 minutes or more. Strain out the herbs and store the mellite away for use.

Storage

Store your ointments, unguents, and mellites in a cool, dark, dry place. Light and warmth break down herbs and natural products, so store them in amber colored jars or cover the jars with paper. Use your products up immediately as long storage also has a negative effect. And after all the purpose here is *fresh*, natural products, isn't it?

II

BASIC
COSMETIC
PLANTS
AND OTHER
NECESSARIES

Basic Cosmetic Plants and Eatables

THE CHOICE OF the following plants was made somewhat subjectively—I *like* them and use them often. One may dispute my selection and argue that it is loose and incomplete; but the plants were carefully chosen for a maximum of uses and they are easily available either fresh or dried. They may be grown in most herb gardens, in pots indoors, or can be found dried in the herb section of your local health food store and in herb stores all over the country. The other natural ingredients in this list, including Honey and Yogurt, are best obtained from health and natural foods stores. The double-starred plants (**) are the five most important plants represented, the single-starred (*) are among the ten most important.

ALMOND—oil and meal

ALOE*—the fresh gel or bottled juice

BENZOIN—as tincture of Benzoin; dried and powdered

CAMOMILE**—flowers; whole or powdered; fresh or dried

CITRUS—peel, fruit or flowers; fresh or dried; pieces or powdered; especially the Orange and the Lemon

CLOVER, RED—flower heads; fresh or dried, powdered or whole

COMFREY**—the root either fresh or dried, in pieces or whole; the leaf either fresh or dried, cut up or powdered

GARLIC**—the cloves; used fresh

GINSENG—the root; dried and powdered

HONEY

LAVENDER*—the flower buds; fresh or dried

LICORICE—the root; dried, powdered or pieces

MARIGOLD**—the flower heads; fresh or dried, whole, pieces or powdered

MINTS—the leaves of all species, but especially the Spearmint (white mint) or the Peppermint (black mint); fresh or dried, whole pieces

NETTLE—the leaves; dried, pieces

ORRIS—the root; dried, pieces or powdered

PANSY OR VIOLET—the flowers or leaves; dried or fresh, whole pieces or powdered

PARSLEY*—the leaves and stem; fresh or dried, whole, powdered or pieces

ROSE*—the leaves, buds or blossoms; fresh or dried, whole, pieces or powdered; also the essential oil and the distilled water

ROSEMARY**—the leaves of flowers; fresh or dried, whole, pieces or powdered

SAGE—the leaves or flowers; fresh or dried, whole, pieces or powdered

SEA PLANTS—all types and varieties of the pods and stripes; fresh or dried, pieces or powdered

STRAWBERRY—the leaves and fruit; fresh or dried, whole or pieces

THYME—the leaves; fresh or dried, whole or powdered

WITCH HAZEL*—the leaves or bark; fresh or dried

YOGURT

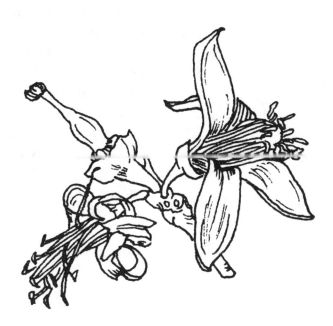

Other Necessaries

ITEM	WHERE AVAILABLE
Beeswax	Hobby shops where candle makings are available
Eggs, Salt,	Grocery store
White kid gloves	Department store
Apple Cider vinegar	Grocery store
Witch Hazel extract	Drug store
HERBS	Herb store, Health food store, or your own garden
Tincture of Benzoin	Drug store
Small postal scale	Stationery store
Cheesecloth	Fabric or grocery store
Muslin	Fabric store
Wire sieve	Grocery, Hardware or Department store
Small funnel	Grocery, Hardware or Department store
Castile soap	Herb store
Chlorophyll	Health food store
Egg beater or wire whip	Grocery, Hardware or Department store
Small enamel pots or double boiler	Grocery, Hardware or Department store
Small enamel bowls	Grocery, Hardware or Department store

Some Approximate Equivalents

	HOW PREPARED*	OUNCES	GRAMS
1 cup *Orange peel*	CS	3 oz.	80 grams
Lemon peel	CS	2	60
Comfrey leaf	CS	1½	45
Comfrey root	CS	6¼	190
Comfrey leaf	PO	3½	100
Comfrey root	PO	3½	100
Lavender buds	WH	1½	40
Rosebuds	WH	1	30
Ginseng	PO	4½	130

Metric Conversions

¼oz	=	7g	4oz	=	115g
½oz	=	15g	6oz	=	170g
1oz	=	30g	½lb	=	225g
2oz	=	55g	¾lb	=	340g
3oz	=	85g	1lb	=	455g

This book was originally published in the United States and, consequently, some units of measurement may be unfamiliar to United Kingdom and Commonwealth readers. To assist, the following conversions are provided:

1 U.S. pint = 16 fl oz (1 Imperial pint = 20 fl oz)

1 U.S. quart = 32 fl oz

1 U.S. cup = 8 fl oz (1 Imperial cup = 10 fl oz)

To measure an American cupful, fill to 8 fl oz on a measuring jug.

*Note: You will notice that after the dried herbs there is a notation, either CS, WH, or PO. These abbreviations are designations for the form in which you may buy herbs. The words are never written out in either catalogs or in the stores, but they mean the following: CS is cut and sifted; WH means the whole form; PO means powdered and GR means ground up. So whenever you go shopping by mail or on foot to your local herb store know also the form in which you wish to purchase the herb.

Flower Scented Oil for the Hair

Salad Oil, Oil of Sweet Almonds, and *Oil of Nuts,* are the only ones used for scenting the hair.

Blanch your Almonds in Hot Water, and when dry, reduce them to powder; sift them through a fine Sieve, strewing a thin layer of Almond–powder, and one of Flowers, over the bottom of the Box lined with Tin. When the box is full, leave them in this situation about twelve hours; then throw away the Flowers, and add fresh ones in the same manner as before, repeating the operation every day for eight successive days. When the Almond-powder is thoroughly impregnated with the scent of the Flowers of choice, put it into a new clean Linen Cloth, and with an Iron Press extract the Oil, which will be strongly scented with the fragrant perfume of the Flower.

—From *The Toilet of Flora,* 1779

III
RECIPES AND A BIT OF HERBAL LORE

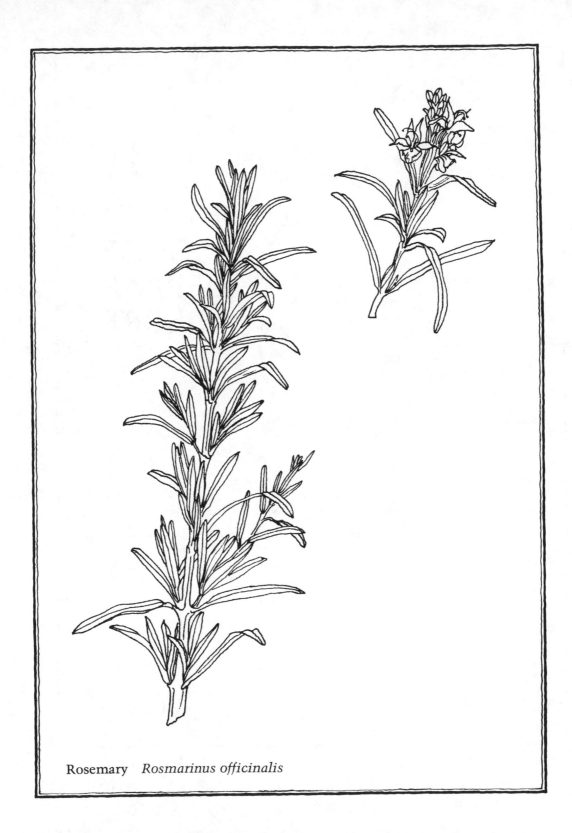

Rosemary *Rosmarinus officinalis*

Rosemary

ROSEMARY IS A BUSHY or trailing plant that grows best near the sea. It takes its name from *ros marinum* or sea dew. It is one of those plants used for hundreds nay thousands of years by many cultures and probably originated in the Mediterranean area. The ancient Romans used the Rosemary for ceremonial, decorative, medicinal and culinary purposes.

Rosemary was burned and used to purify a house of evil or harmful spirits. Not too long ago there were some strange people in the building where I lived. Many fearful happenings were heard in their apartment. When they left I wandered around there cleaning up. I was constantly fearful, I felt there were ghouls and spooks looking over my shoulder. These feelings intimidated me so much that I set a pan of Rosemary and water boiling on the stove, put Rosemary on all the heater ducts, used Rosemary in a pot as incense and carried it through the place as a censor. It took two days for the Rosemary to completely eradicate the evil emanations from the floor and walls!

Rosemary is the herb of remembrance, and an infusion drunk daily is said to improve the memory. The Romans believed that the odor could preserve dead bodies from putrifying. It was used during the days of the Plague to protect wearers from this dread disease.

Now we use Rosemary tea to enliven iced tea, Rosemary charcoal to brush and cleanse teeth, as a tonic, milk facial or body astringent; internally to cause a gentle opening and sweating, and as a growth stimulant on the hair. The scent of Rosemary oil is inhaled to relieve headaches. The oil is applied to the hair roots as a conditioner, or the infusion applied as a hairwash, as it seems to stimulate the hair follicles to renewed activity. From 200 pounds of the flowering tops about 1 pound of oil (wholesale price approximately $9.75) can be obtained.

Protein Herbal Castile Shampoo For Dark Hair

INGREDIENTS:

1 T *Sage* or 6 *leaves* if fresh

2 T *Rosemary* or a goodly pinch
  if fresh

2 T *Irish Moss*, dried

1 T *Nettle*, dried

1 T *Peppermint* or a goodly
  pinch if fresh

1 T *Red Clover* or pinch if fresh

2¼ C *Water*

2 oz. *Castile soap*

A few drops Scent *(Essential
  Oil* of your choice, such
  as *Peppermint* or *Orange)*,
  that has been dissolved in
  ¼ oz. *Tincture of Benzoin*

QUANTITY: Makes about 16 shampoos for short hair or about 12 for long hair.

TO MAKE: Mix the herbs together and boil them with the water in a small enamel pot for 5 minutes or so. Turn off the heat and let the mixture steep. In the meantime, measure out 2 oz. dry Castile soap on a postal scale and put this into an enamel bowl. Strain out the herbs through cheesecloth, silk or muslin and add the herbs to your potted plants or to your bath as fertilizer to plants or body. Add the hot herbal liquid (now about 16 oz. after being boiled and strained) to the soap and beat gently with an egg beater or a wire whisk until the soap is dissolved. You might need to heat the liquid soap a bit to dissolve every bit of it. Place the Herbal Protein Shampoo into a quart container and add the scent. Shake gently. The shampoo is now ready for use.

TO USE: If you are apt to use too much shampoo in the hopes that suds make for a clean head, then take 2 oz. of your Herbal Shampoo and place in a cup with about 4 oz. of water and proceed to wash your head as usual.

TIP: A fine quality Castile soap is available for a very reasonable sum through Indiana Botanic, Hammond, Indiana.

Herbal Castile Shampoo for Light Hair

INGREDIENTS:

2 T *Aloe gel** fresh from
  the cut leaf (optional)
½ C *Camomile*, dried
  or fresh
¼ C *Orange peel*, dried
  or fresh
½ C *Marigold* (Calendula),
  dried or fresh

¼ C *Orris root*
4½ C *Water*
4 oz. *Castile soap*
A few drops *Essential
  Oil*, your choice,
  dissolved in ½ oz.
  Tincture of Benzoin

QUANTITY: This makes 1 quart of shampoo, probably enough for a family of four for 6 weeks if each member shampoos once every 5-8 days.

TO MAKE: Mix together the herbs and water and simmer in a small enamel pot for 5-10 minutes. Turn off the heat and let steep for 10-15 minutes or more while you prepare the other ingredients. In the meantime, measure 4 oz. of dry Castile soap or powder on your postal scale and put this into a 1½ quart enamel bowl. Strain out and discard the herbs somewhere where they can be useful. In a blender, add 1 cup of the strained herbal liquid to the Aloe gel, and blend on low speed until completely integrated. Now add the rest of the quart of herbal liquid to the soap in the bowl and beat with a whisk until the soap is dissolved. Add the blender liquid. You may need to heat the mixture a little to totally dissolve the soap. Pour the shampoo into a quart container, add the scent, shake a bit. If the bottle is not filled to the quart mark, add cold water.

---

*Aloe gel is the clear, translucent sap of an Aloe leaf. To get it, break off a section of leaf, peel off the dark green skin and use the gel.

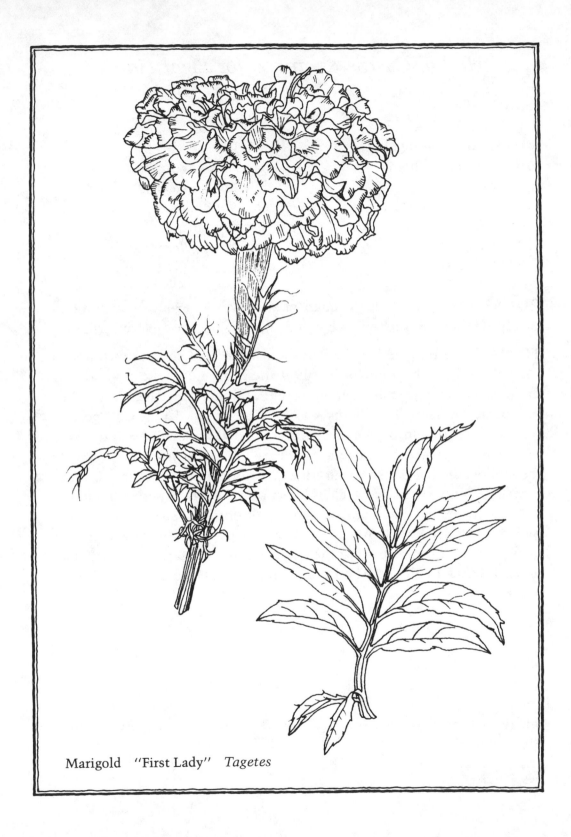

Marigold "First Lady" *Tagetes*

Marigold
(Also Known as Calendula or Tagetes)

CHARLES SKINNER in his *Myths and Legends of Flowers*, 1913, speaks of the Marigold as a flower chosen to express jealousy and fawning.

> In one legend it [Marigold] is a girl who, consumed with envy of a successful rival in the affections of a young man, lost her wits and died.

So if you send someone a Marigold in the language of flowers you are expressing your feelings of jealousy. The Mexican Marigold, *Tagetes*, signifies with its reddish petals the blood of the Aztecs put to death by Spaniards in their lust for land and gold.

The Marigold is one of the most important herbal remedies for babies. When ground up it is used as a body powder; the infusion can be used in the bath to cleanse the skin, as an eyewash, or internally for a soothing draught. It was once used as a drink for young children with the measles. I find the Marigold is best mixed with Camomile and Comfrey as an all purpose super herbal mixture that can be used in creams, oils, ointments, eye lotions, drinks, unguents for any person and especially babies, young children, and those with sensitive skin.

Chopped Marigold flowers are often added to soups for a deliciously distinct flavor. The powder mixed with salt is scattered on meat or the small flowers are added whole to salads that are dressed with oil and vinegar.

Herbal Conditioning Vinegar Rinse for Light Hair

These herbs may be used fresh or dry, whole, or cut and sifted.

INGREDIENTS:

1 C *Marigold flowers*

1 C *Camomile flowers*

½ C *Orange peel*

½ C *Lemon peel* (for oily hair)

½ C *Comfrey root*

2 qts. *Apple cider vinegar*

QUANTITY: Bottle the Herbal Vinegar in 2 one-quart containers.

TO MAKE: Mix all the above herbs together. They can be freshly picked, dried, or a combination of both. Place the herbs in a wide-mouth gallon jar. Heat the vinegar and pour it over the herbs. Cap the jar and shake vigorously and put the jar away in a cool dark place for 10 days. Every day, shake the jar. At the end of the 10 days, strain the herbs out through cheesecloth or silk, pressing the herbs gently to extract most of the vinegar.

TO USE: Use this vinegar on your hair to neutralize the alkalinity of most Castile Shampoos. Mix 2 tablespoons of the Herbal Vinegar with 1 cup warm water and pour over and through clean, wet, just-shampooed hair. Then rinse with clear, cool water.

TO USE ON SALADS: Simply substitute this Herbal Vinegar for any vinegar that you normally use as a salad dressing.

TIP: Remember that dried herbs are about one-half the weight of an equal volume of fresh herbs since the fresh plants lose considerable moisture as they dry. One ounce of freshly picked herbs when dried weighs approximately ¼ to ½ ounce; or 1 cup fresh equals ¼ to ½ cup dry.

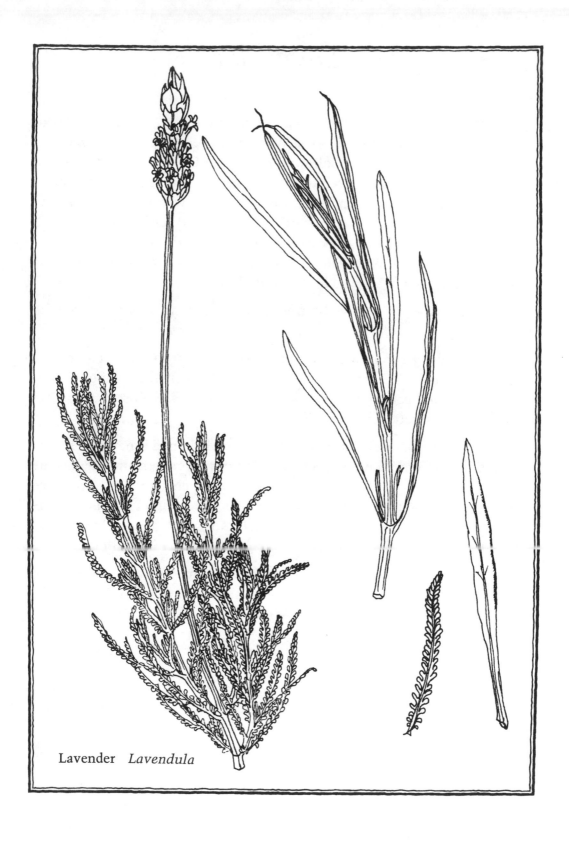

Lavender *Lavendula*

Lavender

As THE ROSEMARY is the *Spirit,* so Lavender is the *Soul,* or according to an old proverb, as a Man is to a Woman. Rosemary and Lavender as messengers from the stars followed Adam and Eve from Paradise in the form of plants as a God-given token to remind this first man and woman of their starlit home. Ever since, they have followed man wherever he goes, through temptations and sickness, and God has given these two lowly plants the power to bestow on man strength, health, endurance, and resistance to disease. Their mission is to follow man until he returns to his starry home. So goes a beautiful old legend.

These two plants have been with us for so long that their origin is indeed lost in antiquity.

Lavender Flowers are used in all types of cosmetics, at home or commercially. The fragrant oil is distilled for use in toilet water, aftershave and perfumery. In the home Lavender and Rosemary oil are used as a first-rate hair conditioner.

My Lavender is currently blooming in its light and limey soil. In two years it has formed an enormous bush with flowers terminating on the ends of eighteen-inch long stems. There is not enough sun to produce intensely fragrant flowers but the fragrance is there and I use the flowers in facial steams, in baths, in teas as a relaxant, in massage oils to revive tired muscles, in shampoos and hair rinses, and dried in potpourris.

I also use Lavender oil in hot footbaths, mixed with water as an underarm deodorant, in small ampules as a reviving inhalant, and directly applied to insect bites or stings.

Lavender / Rosemary Hair Oil

INGREDIENTS:

1 oz. *oil of Rosemary*
⅛ oz. *oil of Lavender*

QUANTITY: Enough for about 6 months of use.

TO MAKE: Simply mix the two oils together and store in the dark or in a small amber or light-proof bottle.

TO USE: Put a few drops of the oil on your palm, brush your palm against your hairbrush and then brush your hair.

TIP: *Proper Hair Brushing:* Every day, rain or shine, men and women should thoroughly brush the hair. Brushing dislodges dirt and distributes the natural hair oils. Bend at the waist (this increases circulation to the scalp) and massage the scalp with fingertips. Then brush hair starting at the nape of the neck with long easy strokes from nape to ends. Follow each of the brush strokes with your other hand to eliminate static electricity. Brush about 100 strokes in this upside down position. This is guaranteed to give new life to your hair.

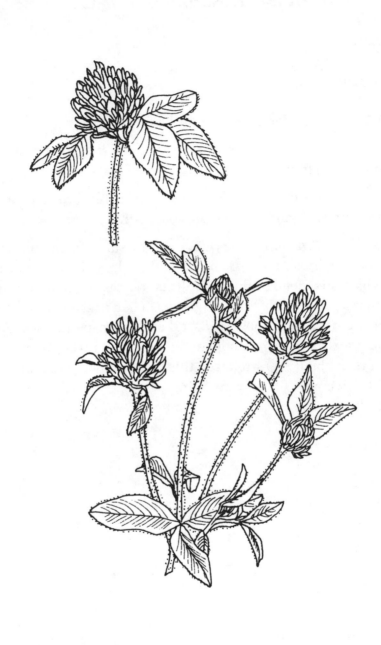

Red Clover   *Trifolium pratense*

Red Clover

The flowers were sad and very still
The night Christ died upon the hill,
Only the clover turned about
And wove green fingers in and out
About the cross. Christ did not see
The clover's little sympathy,
But God looked down, and on each leaf
He marked a tiny sign of grief . . .
A little poignant drop of red
In memory of my son, God said.
    —Anonymous

A BLISSFUL "HONEYEDMOON" TRIP across the desert and over the Rockies took us on a long and steep grade up a four-lane highway. The smoke and pollution from many trucks and cars was so sickening that we pulled over onto a broad grassy shoulder and sat talking for a bit. The wind changed and a delicious smell of honey wafted past. I puzzled over the source, the fragrance itself being immediately recognizable as *Trifolium pratense*, the Red Clover. It was sweet and delicious and a welcome change from exhaust smell, but it took some time to find the plants which were scattered and stunted.

Red Clover with its spot of red on the three-lobed leaf is especially useful for respiratory problems, as a soak for athlete's foot, as a wash for an itchy scalp or as a conditioner for the skin.

Beverage Tea to Improve the Hair Health

INGREDIENTS:

1 T *Red Clover*
1 T *Comfrey leaf*
1 T *Ginseng*
1 T *Spearmint*

1 T *Parsley*
1 T *Rosemary*
1 T *Kelp, Seaweed*
   or *Dulse**

QUANTITY: Makes enough for 8 small pots of tea.

TO MAKE: Use only dried herbs and mix them all together. Store away in a small light-proof container.

TO USE: Every day as often as you like, brew up a cup or a pot of tea. Bring 10 oz. of water to a rolling boil. To the prewarmed teapot, add 1-3 teaspoons of the mixed herbs and 1 teaspoon of Clover Honey. Pour the water over the herbs and honey. Cover the teapot and steep for 3-5 minutes. Strain. Drink.

TIP: Remember that the longer you steep herbs, the more of their properties are released into the water, and consequently the stronger the tea will taste. If you want a mild beverage, steep only 3 minutes or less. If you want healthy hair, steep 10 minutes and drink 4-6 cups per day.

---

*See page 113 for more on sea plants.

KITCHEN COSMETICS

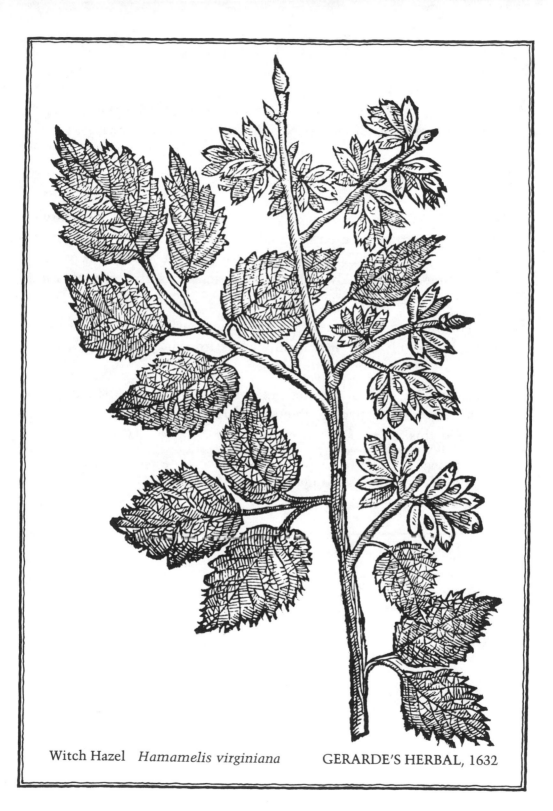

Witch Hazel *Hamamelis virginiana*   GERARDE'S HERBAL, 1632

Witch Hazel

A PLANT WITH a long history of use in witchcraft, the Witch Hazel's branching stems are often used to divine water where there is no known water. The soft, bright green leaves taste rather bitter and slightly aromatic.

Witch hazel is an important and popular plant. An extract of it has been made and sold commercially in the United States for a century or more. This extract is used externally as a scalp rub for dandruff, an astringent wash for inflamed skin, a moist poultice for varicose veins, a general household remedy for burns, cuts, scratches, itches, bites, stings and whatever else you may imagine.

The herb, dried or fresh, is used generously in many cosmetics especially for oily skin. It is mainly an astringent and the decoction is used as a face wash or in bath herbs.

Either the bark or the herb may be used in cosmetics, the bark having the stronger effect. Culbreth, *Materia Medica and Pharmacology*, 1927, has this to say of its properties:

> Astringent, hemostatic, styptic, sedative, tonic; external inflammations, congestion, sore throat (gargle), hemorrhages of nose, uterus, gums; piles, tumors, diarrhea.

Herbal Hair Rinse
For All Types of Hair

INGREDIENTS:

½ C *Rosemary*

½ C *Red Clover*

½ C *Nettle*

and

½ C *Sage* (for dark hair)

or

½ C *Camomile* (for light hair)

or

½ C *Witch Hazel*, leaf or

bark (for oily hair)

or

½ C *Marigold* (for dry hair)

QUANTITY: Makes 2 cups of Herbal Hair Rinse, enough for 4-8 after-shampoo rinses.

TO MAKE: Mix together the dried herbs and store in a covered, light-proof container.

TO USE: Before you shampoo, take ¼ to ½ cup of the herbs and add to 2 cups of water in an enamel pot. Cover the pot, bring to a slow boil, simmer for a few minutes, remove from the heat, and proceed to shampoo your hair. After the last rinse, strain the herbs from the pot, add enough cold water to the herbal brew to be comfortable to your scalp and proceed to rinse your hair. Catch the drippings in the pot and keep pouring them through your hair until they are all used. You may now either rinse your hair with clear water or omit rinse.

TIP: For shiny glossy hair and a minimum of tangles, dry your hair in the sun, wave it about in the breeze, but do *not* touch your hair with comb or brush until it is completely dry. Then, gently pull hair strands apart with fingers and bend over and brush it glossy with a natural-bristle brush.

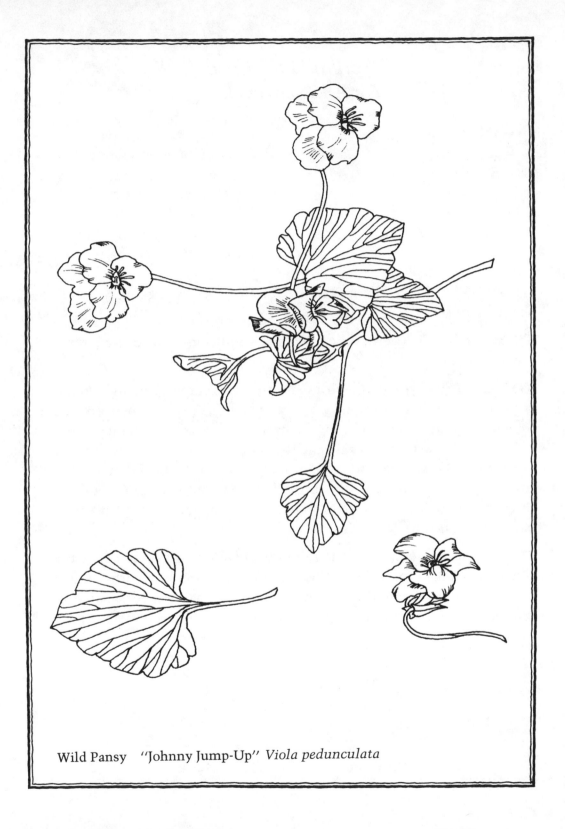

Wild Pansy "Johnny Jump-Up" *Viola pedunculata*

Pansies and Violets

ALL PANSIES ARE really Violas, but not all Violas can be called Pansies. Modern Pansies were developed from two lines of wild Violets in Britain, the *Viola lutea* and *Viola tricolor*. The delicate, simple, fragrant plant we know as the Violet is *Viola odorata*. This Viola, the sweet Violet, has been with us for thousands of years and the Roman naturalist Pliny spoke of it thusly:

> Of Violets, there be some wild and of the field: others domestical, and growing in our gardens. The purple Violets are refrigerative and do coole. And therefore a good liniment is made of them to be applied unto an hot stomacke, against burning inflammations. A frontal likewise may be made of them to be laid unto the forehead. But a peculiar vertue they have besides to stay the running and waterie eyes: Garlands being made of Violets and let upon the head, revive the heaviness of the head, and withstand the overturning of the braines upon over-liberal drinking . . .

He goes on to mention other uses for Violets, some of which were and are: For growths or diseases of the face and neck such as eczema, psoriasis, swollen neck glands, inflamed eyes, pimply complexions. The herb and flowers are used either fresh or dried, either internally or externally, whatever is indicated.

Some modern studies of these plants show that they have a very high content of salicylic acid (a relative of aspirin), iron, Vitamin C and Vitamin A.*

To cook with Violet or Pansy flowers, pick them when the dew has dried but before the sun has baked away all of their fragrance. They can be tossed directly into or onto salads; or to garnish desserts; the leaves can be used as an edible base to molded salads or dips; candied and added to pastries as decorations (mighty delicious this way); to flavor syrup or Honey; or steeped in Honey and applied to the face as a moisturizing stimulant to the circulation.

---

*Violet leaves, according to Euell Gibbons' study, contain 83% water, 210 mg/100 g ascorbic acid, 8258 I.U./100 g Pro-vitamin A.

Herbal Dandruff Rinse

INGREDIENTS:

½ C *Pansy, Violet
    leaves* or *flowers*
½ C *Red Clover*

½ C *Peppermint*
½ C *Nettle*

QUANTITY: Makes 2 cups of Herbal Dandruff Rinse or enough for 4-8 after-shampoo rinses.

TO MAKE: Mix together the dried herbs and store in a covered light-proof container. Then follow the same directions as for the Herbal Hair Rinse on page 41.

TIP: Use dried herbs if you wish to make enough to keep for a few shampoos. If you use fresh herbs, make enough rinse for only 1 application. A mixture of dried and fresh herbs may also be used.

Another Simple Dandruff Rinse

To one cup of extract of Witch Hazel (available in any pharmacy), add a pinch each of the following herbs, either fresh or dried: Comfrey root, Rosemary, Nettle and Lavender. Let the herbs steep for 3-5 days until the aromatic Witch Hazel scent has taken on the more fragrant scent of Rosemary and Lavender. Strain out the herbs. Use the liquid directly. It can be massaged into a clean scalp or used daily as a scalp rub before bedtime. This same liquid is also excellent applied to underarms as a deodorant.

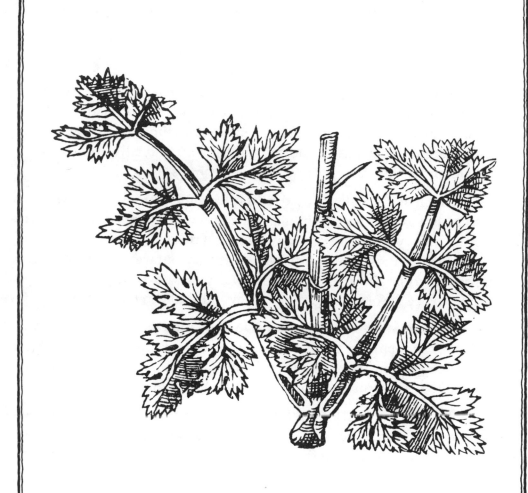

Parsley   *Petroselinum crispum*   PARADISI IN SOLE, 1629

Parsley

Parsley must always be sown on Good Friday.

Parsley should not be transplanted, it means a death in the family.

The reason that parsley is so long appearing after sowing is that, before it sprouts, the roots go down to the Devil.

So GO THREE of the superstitions concerning Parsley, a plant so long in cultivation that neither its wild form is known nor its native habitat. Parsley has an extensive culinary use, in sauces, soups, omelets and in the United States mainly as an uneaten garnish. Nutritionally, it is useful for its content of Vitamins A and C, and of enzymes.

Medicinally, Parsley is used for its cleansing action on the excretory system. It is a diuretic and stimulates the action of the kidneys. It is said to prevent kidney stones if frequently eaten or if the juice is drunk. A chew of Parsley 15 minutes before eating will greatly encourage one's appetite and assist digestion. Frequent eating of Parsley is said to make the nerves strong; hence the old saying: "Eat Parsley and you won't lose your nerve."

Cosmetic values are also extensive; they include pressing fresh juice of Parsley and applying to blemishes and acne or mixing it with cold cream as a healing lotion. The fresh juice or a portion of the bruised plant can be applied to insect stings and bites for immediate relief.

Oil of Parsley is used almost exclusively to flavor commercial food products. It is produced mainly in France by steam distillation of the ripe fruit and is considered toxic by some authorities. In perfumery it is used to obtain a "spicy" or "warm" aroma.

Detoxify Tea For All Conditions
Including a Scruffy Scalp

Parsley is one of several ingredients in this tea, which also includes a variety of herbs not generally mentioned in this book. But I feel that it has an importance belying its seeming simplicity. The tea is used when dieting, instead of liquid when fasting, to improve the all-over health of the body or the hair (drink it instead of other liquids during the day and see how cleansed you will feel). I prefer to have one day a week when I eat very little and drink this mixture, at least one quart a day: It acts as a mild diuretic and body cleanser.

You can purchase this herb tea already made from New Age Creations, San Francisco (see p. 118) or you can easily get the individual ingredients from any herb store and mix them yourself as follows:

USING DRY HERBS	**USING FRESH HERBS**
Can Be Mixed and Stored Away for Later Use	*Must Be Used Immediately*
3 oz. *Parsley*, CS*	1 bunch whole *Parsley*
1 oz. *Celery*, CS	1 pinch chopped *Celery tops*
1 oz. *Fennel seeds*, WH	1 pinch *Fennel seeds*, dried
1 oz. *Cherry stems*, CS or WH	10-15 *Cherry stems*
1 oz. *Dandelion herb*, CS	1 leaf chopped *Dandelion*
1 oz. *Couch grass*, CS	1 pinch *Couch grass*
1 oz. *Corn silk*, WH or CS	1 pinch *Corn silk* from *Red Indian Corn*
1 oz. *Blackberry leaves*, CS	1 *Blackberry leaf*

*See page 23 for a key to abbreviations.

Hair Spray for Fine Hair

INGREDIENTS:
1 *Lemon*
2 C *Water*

QUANTITY: Makes about 1 to 1½ cups of Lemon Hair Spray.

TO MAKE: Chop up the Lemon in a wooden bowl so that you don't lose any of the juice. Add the chopped Lemon to the water in the top of a double boiler. Simmer the mixture until the liquid has been reduced by half. Strain through cheesecloth or fine silk cloth and pour the liquid into a bottle that will fit a pump-type sprayer. A washed and rinsed Windex bottle will do for your spray container. Add ½ cup of water to thin the mixture if necessary.

TO USE: Spray your hair with this mixture whenever necessary. Since it is gentle, with no alcohol or chemical additions, it can be used on children's hair too. Should be made fresh every few days and kept in the fridge between uses.

TIP No. 1:   One cup of the Lemon Hair Spray can be preserved with 1 oz. or more of Bay Rum.

TIP No. 2:   Substitute an Orange for the Lemon for dry hair.

TIP No. 3:   More on Lemon on page 72.

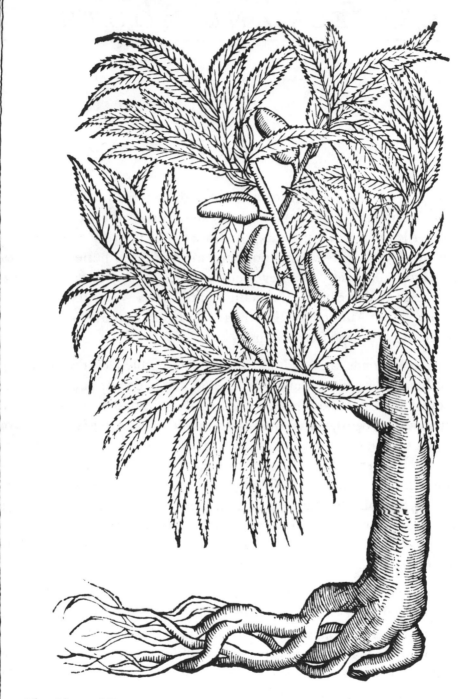

The Almond Tree *Prunus communis* GERARDE'S HERBAL, 1632

Almond

ALMOND MEAL, Almond oil and essence of the bitter Almond are all used in fine cosmetics. As children, it was my sister's and my job to shake down the ripe Almond tree for the nuts which we would then dry, husk, bag, and store. We felt that it was an enormous job and often buried half of our year's crop. Our dad could never quite understand why our seemingly prolific Almond tree had so few pounds of ripe nuts. My sister and I would sell some of our Almonds on the street and my mom would use the rest for food for her body and for her skin.

Ripe Almonds can be ground into a meal in a blender; this meal has a slight bleaching action, and can be used as a skin conditioner and superb smoothing agent. Make a paste by adding the Almond meal to any liquid such as milk, yogurt, water, fruit or vegetable juice. After you clean your face, pat on the Almond paste, allow it to dry, and then wash it off with clear, cool water. Behold the shining clean, smooth result. You can also make *Almond Milk Lotion:* Grind up some fresh Almonds, add a bit of milk, let the mixture stand for 15 minutes, and then strain through fine cheesecloth. The resulting lotion can be used after you wash your face as a fine moisturizing astringent that will combat facial dryness and do a bit of tightening also.

Almond oil makes an excellent all-purpose soothing oil that is used in the making of deliciously fine creams, lotions and body oils. The essence from the Bitter Almond is added to foods to give a nutty taste and Bitter Almond scent that lovers of Christmas cookies know so well, and is also added to cosmetics for a fragrance that reminds students in my Herbal Studies classes of mother and home.

Skin Reviving Face Mask

INGREDIENTS:

1 T *Almond meal*	Some raw *Egg*, beaten
1 T *Marigold*, PO	*Seaweed gel* or *Aloe gel*,
1 T *Camomile*, PO	enough to make a paste

QUANTITY: Several masks.

TO MAKE: Mix all the ingredients together and add a sufficient quantity of the gel to make a thick gooey paste. If it is too fluid, add more Almond meal or herbs and if too thick and gooey, thin with gel or raw egg.

TO USE: Wash your face with warm water and apply a warm water or warm herbal poultice to open the pores. Leave your face (or any other part of your anatomy for that matter) damp dry and apply the mask. Leave the mask on for 10 or more minutes (lie on a slantboard if you have one) while patting it about in upward swirling movements. Then rinse with warm water and follow with a cold water rinse or the Almond Milk Lotion.

WHY: Almond meal is used for smoothing and slight bleaching; Marigold to soothe and heal any facial blemishes; Camomile helps to reduce puffiness; egg helps to replace protein and acts as an emulsifier in this recipe; Aloe is very healing and soothing, while Seaweed is an emollient. Heat opens the pores, the final cold-water rinse closes them, the swirling movements used when applying the mask improve circulation and increase the ability of the skin to release toxins.

TIP: In any recipe such as this it makes sense to set aside some of one's breakfast egg (uncooked) for your healing daily masks. In this way you can stimulate your complexion on a daily basis rather than using the mask only on special occasions.

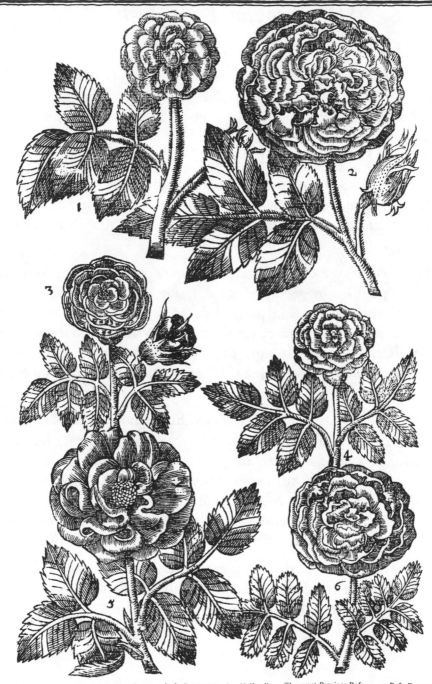

1 *Rofa Damafcena.* The Damaske Rofe.   2 *Rofa Prouincialis fiue Hollandica.* The great Prouince Rofe.   3 *Rofa Franca-furtenfis.* The Franckford Rofe.   4 *Rofa rubra humilis.* The dwarfe red Rofe.   5 *Rofa Hungarica.* The Hungarian Rofe. 6 *Rofa lutea multiplex.* The great double yellow Rofe.

Rose   *Rosa*   PARADISI IN SOLE, 1629

The Rose

Of all flowers Methinks a rose is best.
—Shakespeare

I<small>N</small> *A Discourse on Roses and The Odour of Roses* written by a Mr. Sawer in 1844 we have a history of the discovery of the essence of Roses by the Persians. This discovery is said to have been made in 1612.

> . . . The circumstances attending the discovery are for the first time described in a work written in Persian by Mohammed Achem, entitled *Tarykh Montekheb Lubab,* which is a History of the Great Moguls from 1525 to 1667 . . .

According to the translation, it appears that at the commencement of the marriage of Princess Nour-Djihan with her betrothed, the Princess' mother gave a wedding present of essence of Rosewater and thus we have the first Otto of Rose. A much more delightful history is recounted in the next paragraph where it goes on to say that this marriage fete

> . . . was of a very costly and magnificent character, luxurious amusement of every sort being provided, the princess even carrying her extravagance and prodigality to the extent of causing rosewater to flow through a canal constructed in the flower gardens. It then happened that whilst the emperor and the princess were walking along the bank of this canal they noticed that an oily stratum had concentrated on the rosewater and was floating on its surface; this was carefully collected and recognized by the entire Court as the most delicate of perfumes. What thus resulted from accident was afterwards imitated by art . . .

It is impossible to describe either the beauty of the Rose or its usefulness in just a few short paragraphs. You will find many and varied uses for it in the pages of this book. The Rose petals are used in potpourri or in teas and jellies for their acid astringency. Rosewater is a soothing astringent, Rose hips contain rather large amounts of Vitamin C and some Rose leaves are apple-scented and used in medicinal salves for their healing astringency.

Night-Time Rose Creamy Lotion

INGREDIENTS:

20 fl. oz. *Almond oil*

16 fl. oz. *Rosewater* to
which have been added
1 oz. dried red *Rose
petals*, this soaked for
3 days, then strained
out and removed

3 oz. *Beeswax*

Essence of *Rose*,
if desired

TO MAKE: Into a water bath or the top of a double boiler put the oil and the wax. Heat until the wax is dissolved and then remove pot from the fire. Add the Rosewater slowly, beating all the while, and beat until it is cool. At this point add the essence of Rose a drop at a time, if you like. Beat the creamy lotion until cold, pour into a bottle and store away for use.

TO USE: This lotion makes an excellent Rose Cold Cream to remove old grimy dirt or makeup. Simply apply with clean fingertips and remove with fine tissue. Then you might take a teaspoonful of cornmeal in each palm and rub the hands and face well with it. Rinse with warm water and then cold. Pat the remaining fine film of cream into the skin for night-time smoothing.

WHY: Almond oil and Rosewater as we know is an excellent moisturizing lubricant for normal to dry to sensitive skin; cornmeal is a gentle tonic stimulating to the tissues and acts as a "beauty grain."

TIP: Whenever making fine cosmetics always use a porcelain or glass pot. Some beauty experts recommend stainless steel cooking pots but these often leach poisonous heavy metals into the enclosed liquids. Nonmetal is best for herbs.

Rose Cream for Day Use

INGREDIENTS:

6 fl. oz. *Almond oil*

2 oz. *Beeswax*

1 heaping tsp. anhydrous
   Lanolin

1 tsp. *Borax* dissolved in
   4 fl. oz. *Rosewater*

2 tsp. *Zinc Oxide* rubbed
   into a smooth cream
   with 4 fl. oz.
   Almond oil

10-20 drops *oil of Rose*

QUANTITY: Makes enough for about three 4 oz. cream jars.

TO MAKE: Heat the beeswax and the lanolin gently in a water bath. Do not let the wax simmer or burn. Remove from heat and add the Almond oil slowly. Add the zinc oxide-Almond oil cream beating the mixture continuously. Add the borax-Rosewater and beat until cool. Add enough oil of Rose to scent the mixture to your liking. Beat until cold with a small wooden spoon. Pour into three 4 oz. cream jars and let sit until solidified.

TO USE: This makes an excellent everyday cream that can be used under makeup or as a moisturizer. Simply rub gently onto face, hands or throat. As a throat moisturizer the cream is excellent, especially when rubbed in with a large marble or small avocado pit. Rub in gentle circular motions while looking up into the sky, thereby stretching and stimulating your neck muscles.

WHY: Almond oil replaces necessary body oils; Rosewater is a gentle astringent and moisturizer replacing liquid to the cells and tightening the skin; lanolin is a potent emollient and very much like human oils; borax is a skin softener and will help to produce a very white cream while its disadvantage is that it often adds a grainy texture; zinc oxide is useful for healing reddened, sore or irritated skin.

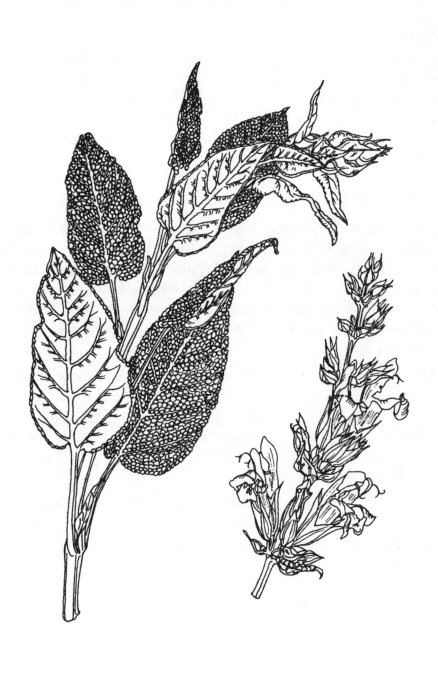

Sage   "Holt Mammoth"   *Salvia*

Sage

"He who wouldst live for aye
Must eat sage in May!"
—Old Proverb

THERE ARE MANY varieties and species of Sage. Some are used for medicine, some for cosmetics and some for aromatherapy. Sage is used as an internal tea and acts as an external deodorant. Its use is opposite that of a diaphoretic, or something that makes you sweat. If you have heavy discharges, whether they be mucus from nose or heavy perspiration from the armpits, then Sage is the herb for you. Sage was regarded by the old herbalists as a panacea for everything just as Ginseng and Garlic are regarded now. Sage cheese* is delicious and was thought to strengthen both mind and muscle. Sage in the bath is a prescription for sore muscles. Sage infusion is good for sore throats; mixed with other herbs it is useful to darken the hair and also helps to cleanse the scalp of dandruff. Sage can be used in facial steams for cleansing, especially for oily skin. I use it mainly in baths and sleep pillows.

Sage Butter

Sage butter is made with a cube of sweet butter. Soften the butter by mashing with a fork. Add 1 or 2 tablespoons of finely chopped fresh Sage. Mash together and use on fresh vegetables or toast wedges.

---

*Sage cheese is made in Great Britain and the USA by crushing fresh sage to get the color and flavour, and adding pieces of chopped Sage for eye appeal. The basic cheese is a white Cheddar.

Rose Hip Honey Facial or Sore Throat Cure

INGREDIENTS:

½ lb. ripe *Rose hips*
  (about 2 heaping cups)
¾ C *Water*

¾ C *Sage Honey*
4 pieces of *candied Ginger*
  (optional)

QUANTITY: Makes 8 or more applications to toast or face.

TO MAKE: Put Rose hips, Ginger and water into an enamel pot and simmer gently. Mash the Rose hips with a potato masher and simmer until the hips are very mushy, about 15 minutes. Strain through cheesecloth or a potato ricer to filter out the Rose seeds. Discard the seeds into your garden or compost heap. Add Sage Honey to Rose hip sauce and boil for a few minutes to half an hour, depending on thickness desired. Pour the Rose Hip Honey into a sterile container and refrigerate.

TO USE: For a moisturizing and soothing facial simply apply a thick layer to your cleaned face. Gently pat face in circular upwards motions until the Rose Hip Honey is tacky. To remove, rinse with warm water and then follow with a stimulating pat of cold water. It would also be nice to leave the Rose Hip Honey on the face and take an Herbal Bath or shower to allow the Rose Honey time to penetrate the pores.

TIP: This syrup may also be used for toast or waffles; or a tablespoonful may be taken every few hours to soothe a sore throat. Very, very tasty!

Healing Cleansing Cream

INGREDIENTS:

4 oz. *Almond oil*

4 oz. pure *Lard* or
   solid *Vegetable Shortening*

1 oz. *Beeswax*

3 oz. *Aloe Vera gel*

QUANTITY: 10 or more applications.

TO MAKE: Melt the beeswax and the Almond oil in a nonmetal pot or the top of a double boiler. Remove from the fire, add the lard and beat until smooth, then add the gel and beat again until smooth and cold.

TO USE: Simply apply this cream to any sore, burning place or as a night-time emollient or daytime cream under your makeup. This is especially useful to actors who have to use heavy layers of makeup and have often become sensitized to them.

WHY: The juice and the gel of the Aloe Vera have been used throughout the ages, in many lands and by many people for any sore, irritated surface, internally or externally, especially for irritations associated with heat.

TIP: Aloe Vera juice is bottled by Aloe Products in Hunt, Texas and available by mail order through them or through most health stores. You may also obtain the gel by simply scraping out the inside of a large fat Aloe leaf and putting it into a blender. The gel liquefies and may be added as juice to any cosmetic recipe.

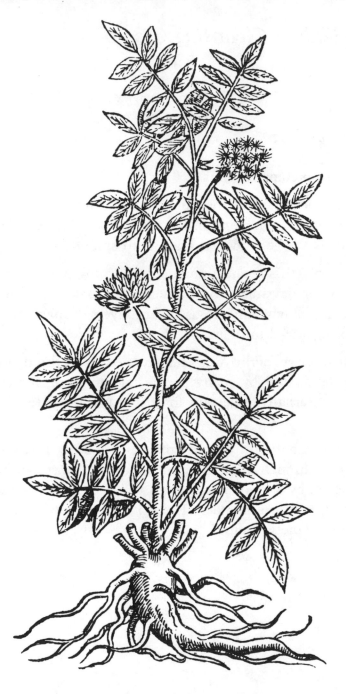

Licorice   *Glycyrrhiza glabra*   PARADISI IN SOLE, 1629

Licorice

OH HOW WE LOVE the Licorice for its relaxing effect on the pores when used in the steam cleaning mixture; and we chew on the root to soothe and heal a sore throat. Some like to drink Licorice root tea although it is much too strong for my taste. Culpeper gives a dandy recipe for Licorice:

> Juice of Liquorice simple. Infuse Liquorice Roots cleansed and gently bruised, three days in Spring Water, so much that it may over-top the roots the breadth of three fingers, then boil it a little, and press it hard out, and boil the liquor with a gentle fire to its due thickness. It is vulgarly known to be good against coughs, colds, etc. and a strengthner of the lungs.

Homemade Toothpaste

INGREDIENTS:

1 tsp. dried *Irish Moss*

1 C *Water*

1 tsp. *Salt*

1 tsp. *Baking soda*

A few drops *Chlorophyll* (available in a pharmacy, or health food store)

2 drops *oil of Licorice, Fennel* or *Anise*

TO MAKE: Soak the moss in the water for about 15 minutes and then bring it to a slow boil in your small enamel pot and *simmer* for 10-15 minutes. The moss may or may not completely dissolve. In any case, strain the gel through cheesecloth into a small container. Mix salt and soda and add to the gel, incorporating it completely. Add chlorophyll and Licorice oil and mix completely.

TO USE: Brush as usual, using only a small amount.

Herbal Steam Cleaning

INGREDIENTS:

Oily Skin or Large Pores

1 T *Comfrey leaf*, CS
2 T *Lavender flowers*
3 T *Licorice root*, PO
1 T *Lemon peel* or *leaf*, CS
1 T *Peppermint*, CS or WH
1 T *Pansy*, CS or WH
1 T *Parsley*, any way
1 T *Rosebud* or *leaf*, any way
1 T *Strawberry leaves*

Dry or Itchy Skin

2 T *Comfrey leaf*, CS
1 T *Comfrey root*, CS
3 T *Licorice root*, PO
2 T *Camomile flowers*, WH
1 T *Red Clover heads*
1 T *Pansy*, CS or WH
1 T *Ginseng*, PO
1 T *Kelp, Dulse* or *Irish Moss*, CS

QUANTITY: Makes 4-6 steams.

TO MAKE: Mix all the dried herbs together and store away for later use. About once or twice a week, whenever you think necessary, put 2-4 tablespoons of the herb mixture into a tall, narrow enamel or glass pot and add 2-3 cups of water. Cover the pot and bring to a boil and simmer gently for 3-5 minutes. Remove from heat placing the covered pot on a low table. Allow the herbs to steep for a few minutes.

TO USE: Cover your hair with a towel and remove the lid from the pot. Putting your face over the pot and covering the pot and sides of face with the towel, let the herbal steam relax, cleanse and medicate your pores. You can move your face about in the steam so that it covers every area of your face and neck. You can blow into the water to create more steam. Wipe away the dirt and oil with a clean washcloth, splash warm water on your face and then rinse with cool mineral water to close the pores. Pat dry.

WHY: In the mixture for oily skin, Licorice and Lavender act as a stimulant to the pores to normalize their action, Rose and Lemon function as astringents, Comfrey and Pansy serve as healing herbs and Lavender, Peppermint, Parsley and Strawberry act as alteratives to restore more normal function to the sebaceous glands. In the mixture for dry skin, Comfrey and Pansy are healing; Licorice relaxes the pores; Camomile and Clover soothe; Parsley and Ginseng unclog pores, and act as an emollient.

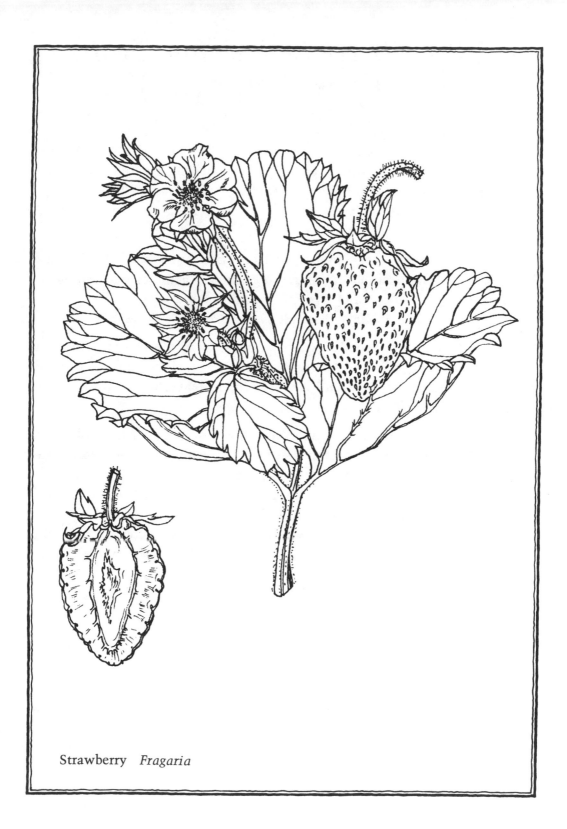

Strawberry *Fragaria*

Strawberry Leaves and Fruits
And Other Berries as Well

IN THE ELIZABETHAN LANGUAGE of flowers, the berry of the strawberry means either "Intoxication and Delight," "You are delicious," "Good Luck Gift to a Woman," "Perfect Righteousness," or is "Symbolic of a righteous man whose fruits are good works." The Strawberry leaves are symbols of "perfection and completion."

Strawberry leaves contain four times more Vitamin C than Orange juice: the relationship is 229 mg/100 g edible portion for the Strawberry and only 50mg/100g for Orange juice, as found in the book, *Composition and Facts About Foods* by Ford Heritage, 1968.

Delicious astringent teas can be made from the leaves of all berry plants that are useful internally for diarrhea; or when applied externally in the form of steam or poultice. Strawberry leaves are used for overactive sebaceous glands.

The Strawberry juice is an excellent addition to creams and lotions for oily or sallow skins. Simply add 1 oz. of freshly squeezed and strained juice to every 4 oz. of cream or lotion that you make. An excellent mask for tired skin is to mash up some fresh Strawberries and mix them with Yogurt and a bit of Almond meal to hold it together. Apply this to your skin and lie down for 1½ hours. You will get up with you and your skin feeling much more refreshed and revitalized. Then simply rinse off the mask with clear water. You can add any berry juice to any of the basic recipes given here. It is simple to tailor-make cosmetics to one's individual needs and complexion.

Facial Conditioning Vinegar Rinse
or
Delicious Salad Vinegar

INGREDIENTS:

1 T *Berry leaves*
5 T *Rose buds* or *flowers*
4 T *Sage leaves*

2 T *Rosemary leaves*
1 C *Apple Cider vinegar*
¾ C *Rosewater*

QUANTITY: Makes up to 20 applications.

TO MAKE: Place the herbs in a crockery or glass jar. Heat the vinegar and then pour it over the herbs. Cap the jar and shake it once a day for 10 days. At the end of this time, strain the liquid through cheesecloth or muslin into another container. Add Rosewater to the herb dregs and shake it about. Strain the Rosewater out and add it to the Herbal Vinegar. Shake, cap, and store away for use.

TO USE: Simply apply to a clean face as an astringent or aftershave lotion or mouthwash or body lotion. It may also be mixed with vegetable oil and used as a tasty salad dressing.

TIP: The strained herbs from these recipes can always be used in the bath to nourish your skin or in the compost pile to nourish the earth.

Rose Eye Wash for Sore, Tired or Irritated Eyes

INGREDIENTS:
1 oz. *Rosewater*
8 oz. *Water*
9 *Rosebuds*

QUANTITY: Makes 3-8 eye or face washes.

TO MAKE: In a small covered enamel pot, bring the Rosebuds and water to a slow boil, lower the heat, remove the cover and simmer for a minute or two until some of the water boils off. Strain out the liquid into a clean container and refrigerate. When cool, add the Rosewater to 4 oz. of the herbal liquid. You must use this liquid within 3 days.

TO USE: Rinse your eyes whenever necessary using this fluid with either an eyecup or the hollow of your palm.

TIP No. 1:   You can also add 1 oz. Rosewater directly to 4 oz. of distilled or boiled water, without using the Rosebuds called for above and bottle the liquid. This will not spoil and may be used at your leisure.

TIP No. 2:   Rosewater may be purchased at any old-fashioned pharmacy, herb or nutrition store and in most fine liquor stores (Rosewater is often used in fine mixed drinks). You might also find it available in Turkish or Middle Eastern speciality shops.

Marigold Face Mask

INGREDIENTS:

1 T *Marigold flowers*   1 T *Carrots,* well-mashed
1 T *Camomile flowers*   1 T *Lecithin granules*
½ C *Water*   1 tsp. *Wheat germ oil*
Almond oil, as much as is necessary

QUANTITY: 1-2 masks

TO MAKE: Bring water to a boil and pour over the Marigold and Camomile flowers. Cover and set aside. Mash the carrots, add wheat germ oil. Strain out the liquid from the flowers and add them to the carrot-wheat germ oil. Mix thoroughly and add the lecithin granules. If you have a blender, blend it finely. The texture can be changed with the addition of Almond oil; add a bit to make a smooth cream for dry skin; if you have oily skin add enough Almond oil to blend these disparate ingredients.

TO USE: Wash face. Steam clean it for a few minutes with one of the steam mixtures. Apply a thick layer of the Marigold Face Mask to the face in smooth upward motions. Rest on a slantboard or rock in a rocking chair, but in any case leave the mask on for 15 minutes. Wipe it off with tissues, rinse with warm water and then close your pores with a refreshing cold water rinse.

WHY: Marigold and Camomile flower infusion is healing to the tissues; carrots add texture and Vitamin A that may or may not be absorbed through the skin; lecithin is an emulsifying agent in the recipe that is also necessary for healthy tissues; wheat germ oil adds Vitamin E; and the Almond oil is for a creamy consistency.

TIP: This mask does not harden but stays relatively moist. It will leave your skin smoother and refreshed, stimulating both facial circulation and muscles.

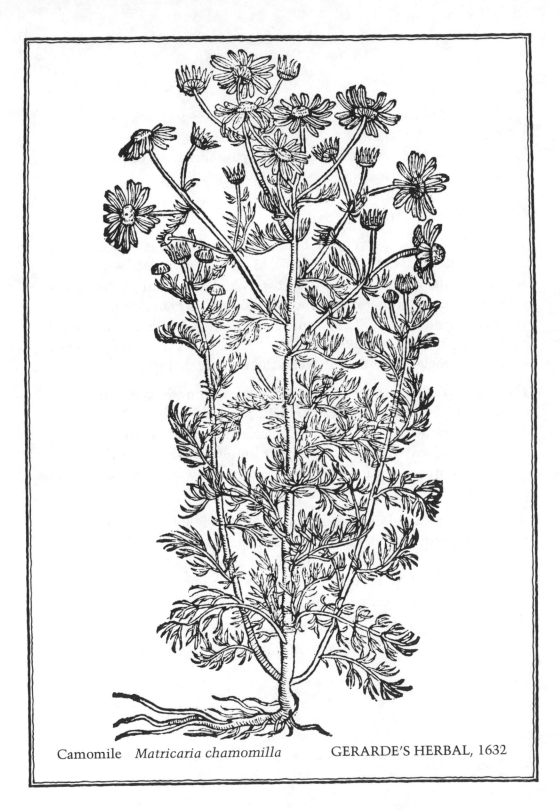

Camomile *Matricaria chamomilla*   GERARDE'S HERBAL, 1632

Camomile
Simple Flower of Beauty

THIS PLANT, a native of western Europe and western North Africa, has a many-branched creeping stem with fragrant, downy, divided leaves. The flower heads are solitary and have white rays and a fragrant yellow center called the disc floret. These flower heads are used either dried or fresh, cosmetically or medicinally. Externally, they will reduce skin puffiness and clean the pores of impurities. An excellent mixture of herbs for the bath and especially for steam cleaning of the skin would be composed of Camomile, Licorice, Comfrey root and maybe a little Mint as an aromatic. Camomile flowers mixed with Poppy heads and simmered in oil make an excellent poultice to reduce external pains from sprains and bruises. A thick concoction of the flowers with Marigolds is excellent as a hair rinse or dye. Camomile infusion taken internally is used for stomach upset or for problem sleepers and externally in the bath to reduce fatigue. It also makes an excellent massage oil for aching muscles. The flowers have been cultivated and in use for over 4500 years.

I love the simple mat-like English Camomile. We use it in place of grass, mow it once a month and take great pleasure in walking on it. With every step a sweet delicious fragrance exudes from the plant that is said to be beneficial to the nervous system.

Underarm Deodorants

INGREDIENTS:

Orange peel, PO

Lemon peel, PO

Orris root, PO

Variation:

Camomile, PO

Marigold, PO

Comfrey root, PO

Variation:

Lavender, PO

Lemon peel, PO

Variation:

Sage, PO

Lemon peel, PO

TO MAKE: Mix together equal quantities of the powdered herbs.

TO USE: Simply pat some of the powder on the offending area, be it underarm or crotch. They are all excellent and effective mixtures for use as deodorants.

TIP: You can also sew up little squares of muslin and stuff them with some of the powder to make aromatic sachets for your drawers and linen closets.

Other Deodorants

INGREDIENTS:

Any Essential *Oil*, 5 drops

½ C *Water*

TO MAKE: In a pump-type spray container or an atomizer, mix the essential oil and water, shake it up each time before use and spray on your body or underarms as a deodorant. Should not be used directly on the genitalia.

TIP: The most effective oils for use as deodorants are the natural oils. Any oil can give an allergic reaction to one who is susceptible, but I have found that synthetic oils affect the skin negatively more often than natural ones. I prefer the following scents: Sage, Lavender, Lemon or Basil.

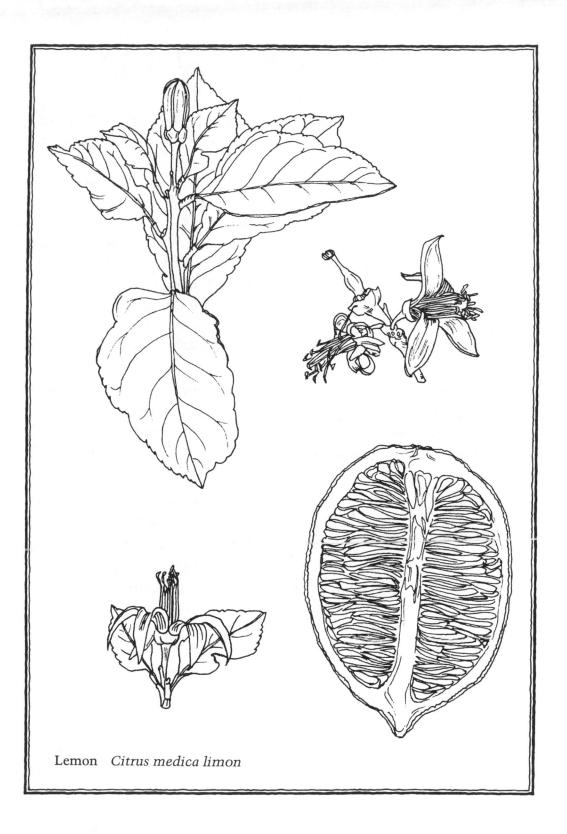

Lemon   *Citrus medica limon*

Citrus–Lemons and Limes

THE HOME OF the Lemon was southeastern Asia before it migrated throughout the world, being brought to the Mediterranean about 1000 A.D. by the Arabs. The Arabs loved the Lemon and used it then and now in many of their national dishes. It was an indispensable item in their cuisine. Originally the Lemon was a medicine rather than a food. Its peel and juice are cooling and are mentioned by Pliny the Elder (the great Roman naturalist) as being used by pregnant women "to stay the flux and the vomit." To those who are inclined to morning sickness, suck on a Lemon before getting out of bed or drink Lemon juice and water. Lemon juice and water is used by fasters and dieters. The Lemon has been used in many types of intestinal disorders, to stop bleeding from wounds, and as a source of Vitamin C. The pectin in Lemon is an important ingredient in jellies.

Lemon is a natural bleach. If you make a thick decoction of Lemon, Camomile and Marigold and apply it to your hair as a pack and sit in the sun for a few hours you can bring golden highlights to dark hair and turn mousey brown hair a golden blond. The Lemon acts as a bleach and the Camomile and Marigold give color.

Lemon is also a natural for the arms and hands. Mixed with oil and used regularly it will protect detergent or roughened hands and the Lemon skins rubbed on elbows will bleach them slightly.

Lemon rind oil, natural and synthetic, is used in perfumery to scent products that range from perfumes to toilet bowls. Lemon blossom oils, as far as I can determine, are rarely if ever used in perfumery.

Lemon Hand Cream

INGREDIENTS:

Almond oil

Beeswax

Lemon juice, freshly squeezed

Lemon oil

TO MAKE: Squeeze a Lemon and strain through cheesecloth. Pour the juice into a measuring cup and add an equal amount of Almond oil. In a small butter melting pot put a thin piece of beeswax. I use approximately 1 teaspoon beeswax for every 3 oz. of cream, this amounts to a *thin* sheet about an inch square. Add to the pot a bit of the Almond oil that has collected above the Lemon juice in the measuring cup. Heat over a medium fire, gently shaking the pot, about 30 seconds or more. Take the pot on and off the fire so that the wax melts but does not burn. Add the rest of the contents of the measuring cup. Heat, shake, and stir with a wooden spoon until the wax has completely melted. Remove from the fire. Stir until cool with the wooden spoon. Add one drop of Lemon oil for every oz. of cream. Give it another stir and transfer to a cream jar or bottle. Cap it. Now shake it every few minutes until the cream is completely cold.

TO USE: Rub a little bit on hands or body whenever necessary.

WHY: This cream is excellent to soften and smooth rough hands. The oil is an emollient, the Lemon is a protectant and texturizer.

TIP: Lemon Hand Cream is so easy to make (and so lengthy to describe) but takes less than 5 minutes, so only make one Lemon's worth at a time. Your measurements then will *probably* be 1½ oz. Lemon juice, 1½ oz. Almond oil, 1 tsp. beeswax, and 3 drops Lemon oil.

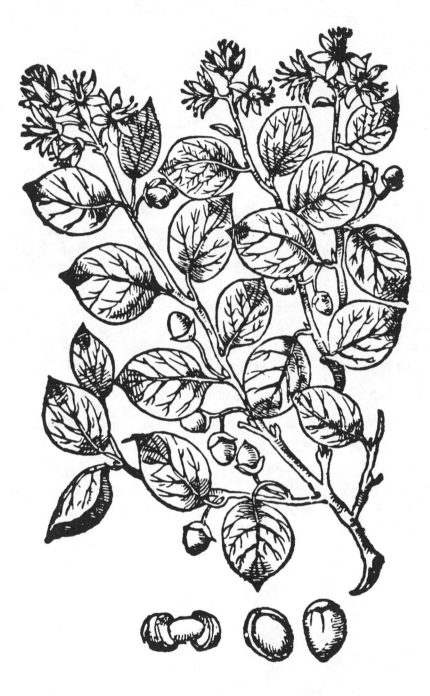

Benzoin *Styrax benzoin*   GERARDE'S HERBAL, 1632

Benzoin—A Plant Resin

*P*ERFUME *and Flavor Materials of Natural Origin*, 1960, by Steffen Arctander has this to say of Benzoin tincture, ". . . used in skin preparations for its skin-healing effect and, occasionally, in certain cosmetic preparations for its antioxidant effect". This basically covers its cosmetic use.

Styrax benzoin is a tree, found in Indochina, whose exudations have been known and used for thousands of years. Historically, the Assyrians used it and it is mentioned in an Assyrian herbal dated 700 B.C. This exudation does not emanate from a normal or healthy tree. Firstly, the tree is wounded to its cambium layer; it then produces ducts that secrete a resin that closes the wound and heals the tree. This resin is the substance known and used as Benzoin.

Benzoin as a solid powder is used in potpourris and solid perfumes as a fixative. When tinctured with alcohol, Benzoin is used as a skin preservative. Years ago, when my Great Dane was getting old and fat, his elbows became raw and hairless from too many years of use and lying down in the sun. We applied tincture of Benzoin as a protective film twice a day to the denuded portion as an antiseptic to keep it free from infection.

A Treatment for Hands

INGREDIENTS:

Soft kid gloves

1 C *Almond meal*

1 T *Comfrey root,* PO

1 T *Parsley,* PO

Some *Honey*

Some *raw Egg*

1 tsp. *Tincture of Benzoin*

QUANTITY: Makes about 12 beautifying hand treatments.

TO MAKE: Mix the herbs and Almond meal together and store away. When your hands need care, take about 2 tablespoons of the herbal mixture and mix in a small bowl with a bit of the morning's egg (before it is cooked of course), the Benzoin, and enough Honey to make a thick but non-drippy goo.

TO USE: About once a month when your hands get dry and chapped or red and rough, pat a thick layer of the goo all over your hands, massaging around each and every finger and then ask someone to put on the gloves for you. Go to bed.

WHY: During the night the Almond will smooth, the Comfrey heal, the Benzoin protect, the Parsley medicate and the Honey will soothe all those problems that your hands have accumulated during the month. Kid gloves are important because they do not absorb the mixture, whereas with cotton gloves the cotton itself absorbs, leaving very little for your hands. The gloves can be washed by hand or in the washing machine after each use.

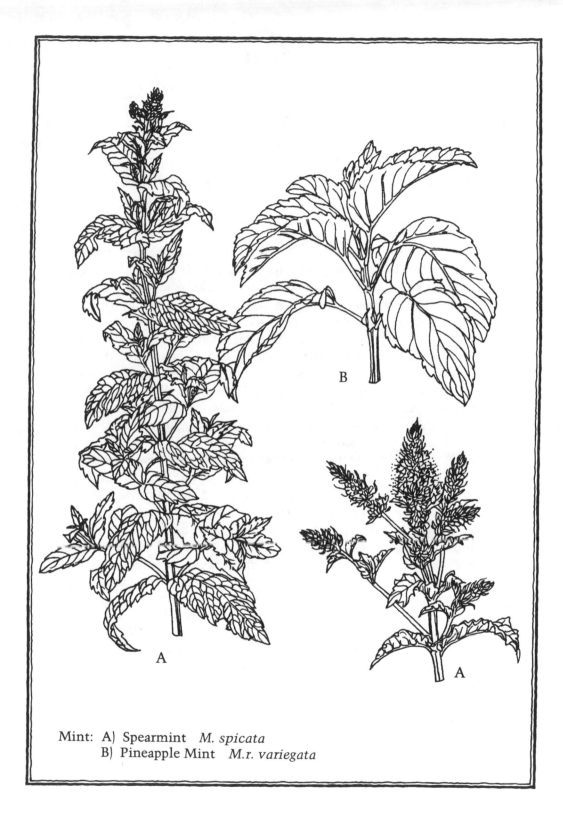

Mint: A) Spearmint *M. spicata*
      B) Pineapple Mint *M.r. variegata*

Mint

THE NAME MINT is English and has been derived from the word Mind; there are many kinds of Mint such as the *Breath* or *Lung Mint, Corn Mint, Spear Mint, Water Mint* and others. Here again we have a genus of plants that has been used for so long and for so many medicinal and cosmetic purposes that the telling would take pages and pages. Instead, I would like to relate to you a lovely myth of the Mint.*

Once upon a time before Man was on the Earth all the creatures of the world lived in harmony and balance with one another. Then came the time when Man was to leave his home, the Kingdom of the Golden Mid-day, and inhabit the Earth. The King of the Kingdom worried about Man and his new home and sent his twin sons to go before Man and make everything right. To his sons, he gave great treasure, strength, and to each a golden disc of *light* and sent them on their way. They met with many adventures. They met the creature with many arms who with his mighty Breath blew them on their way into another Kingdom. They met the lovely Corn Woman who gave them corn to eat and showed them the way to the next country. They met the one who keeps the world in balance and gave one twin a magic Spear and the other a mighty Shield to protect and defend Man with; and then this creature showed them to the great Ocean. Here they met the great Water Bearer who quieted the monstrous waves, and in exchange for showing them the way to Earth he took all their treasures. But he gave the twin sons a magic drink mixed with every sound and color of the waves, and it gave them the power to remember and see clearly forever all their past adventures. By the power of this magic drink the two Bringers of Light from the Land of the Golden Mid-day were transformed into homely plants that stood on earth awaiting the arrival of Man. When Man came he saw the plants and remembered some of his past in the wonderful Kingdom; he smelled the wonderful scents, and pictures of the events of the twins' journeys appeared in his Mind. So whenever Man was asked the name of the plants, he called them Mint.

---

*Adapted from a legend appearing in *Herbs in Nutrition*, 1962, by Maria Geuter.

Lemon Mint Elbow Bleach

INGREDIENTS:

½ C *Mint Water*

½ *Lemon,* squeezed

TO MAKE: Make a thick infusion of Peppermint, strain out the herb and to ½ cup of the liquid add the Lemon juice. Mix together.

TO USE: While studying or working, apply this liquid with cotton pads to the elbows; let it dry and make another application. Repeat applications 3 or 4 times. Do not remove.

WHY: The Lemon juice acts as a bleach, the Mint as a soothing aromatic astringent.

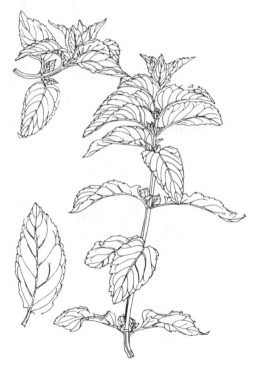

Peppermint   *M. piperita*

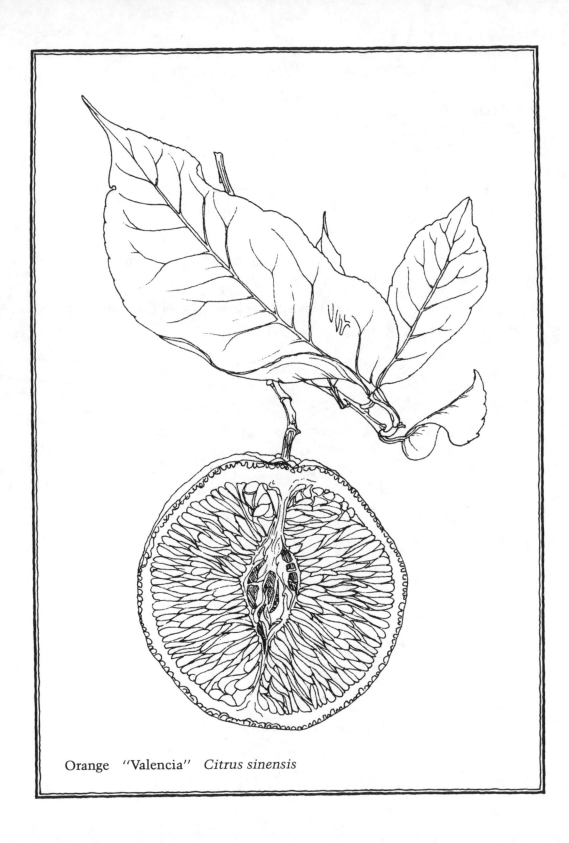

Orange "Valencia" *Citrus sinensis*

Citrus–The Orange

AN ORANGE used for tea, for fragrance in potpourri, or in cosmetic preparations first must be properly prepared. Eat the Orange meat and drink the juice but save the peel. With the back of a knife or your fingers scrape off from the peel as much of the white membranous layer as you can. This membrane contains most of the bioflavonoids and should be eaten. In the peel are the oil glands with most of the Vitamin C. Scrape off this white part and then hang the peel to dry. When it is completely dry, store the peel in a dark container, out of the light and somewhere where it is not damp. A paper bag is a good storage container. The peel is then used in various ways.

Orange peel oil flavors foods and is added to cosmetics, medicines and potpourri. Orange peel is used in herbalism as a tonic to provide Vitamin C and as a flavoring; in cosmetics as a scent and a dry skin application. In hair rinses and shampoos the peel lightens and brightens hair. Orange flower oil is used for cosmetics and to make Orange flower water. A tea of Orange flowers is used as a mild stimulant to the nervous system. The small immature fruits can be put into lingerie drawers for fragrance and into liqueurs for taste.

In Christian art the Orange tree is symbolically regarded as representing purity, generous behavior and a chaste manner. It is often seen in paintings of the Blessed Virgin Mary. Jupiter gave an Orange to Juno when he married her and thus the Orange blossoms that a bride carries are a symbol of marriage.

Citrus Bath Herbs

INGREDIENTS:
Use only dried materials.

1 oz. *Orange peel*, CS

1 oz. *Orange flowers*, WH

1 oz. *Lemon peel*, CS

1 oz. *Comfrey leaves*, CS

1 oz. *Camomile*, WH

1 oz. *Almond meal*

QUANTITY: Makes 6-12 baths.

TO MAKE: Mix together and store away for use.

TO USE: At bath time you may, 1) put a large handful of the mixed herbs into a muslin bag and drop the bag in the hot tub; 2) drop the herbs directly into the water; 3) put the herbs into a perforated metal ball available in the cooking section of department stores and often used in the cooking of rice; 4) make an infusion of herbs and strain the liquid into the tub (see p. 17).

WHY: In this bath mixture, Orange peel soothes the skin, Orange flowers impart fragrance, Lemon peel is an astringent, Comfrey leaves are a healing emollient and astringent, Camomile is soothing and a healer, and Almond meal adds a slippery feel.

TIP: There are several kinds of metal balls used in cooking rice. Some have chains attached that can be hung from the edge of pot or tub. One small 3″ diameter ball I purchased came equipped with a cork float that was perfect in my tub. Now I can always keep track of my bath ball.

How To Make Body Oils

THE EASIEST WAY to make oils that incorporate the qualities of herbs is to put the herbs in the oil for a few days and then strain them out. In practice, however, it is a bit more difficult than this, but not much more.

First, get your herbs together. Buy them already dried or pick and dry the plants according to the directions on page 16. If you have already dried plants, put them into a wide-mouth gallon bottle, about 1 pound of herbs to 1 gallon of oil. The more herbs the stronger the oil. Put them into the bottle and add the oil. I use various mixtures and combinations of oils according to my needs but prefer the mix of equal parts of soy oil, corn oil and sunflower oil. This mixture of oils provides most, if not all of the essential fatty acids and has a nice slippery feel. Many old herbals insist on infusing herbs only in pure olive oil. But feel free to use the oil of your choice. A little practice and experience here will teach you a great deal. The herbs must stay immersed in the oil or mold will occur on whatever floats above the oil.

Infuse the herbs in a nice warm spot for 5-10 days. Then put a funnel lined with cheesecloth into a gallon bottle and strain the oil. Let the oil pass through the cheesecloth naturally. DO NOT squeeze. Now, smell the newly strained oil and add essential oil of your choice that will harmonize with the herbs that you started with.

Depending on the ingredients, this oil can now be used for salads, gentle cooking, as a marinade for meat, for rubbing on bodies, as perfume oil (if scented strongly), as bath oil, or as a cosmetic or medicinal oil.

Almond Kernel Skin Oil

INGREDIENTS:

4 oz. *Almond oil*
A few drops of essential *Oil* of your choice

TO MAKE: Mix the two oils together and store away for use in an amber or light-proof 4 oz. bottle.

TO USE: Use directly on the skin as a face or body oil, or use as perfume.

Perfection Skin Oil

INGREDIENTS:

1 oz. *Soy oil*
1 oz. *Safflower oil*
1 oz. *Wheat germ oil*
3 drops *Orange oil*, essential

1 oz. *Peanut oil*
1 oz. *Corn oil*
1 oz. *Vitamin E*, liquid
3 drops *Lemon oil*

TO MAKE: Simply mix all the above oils together and shake them up. Store in an 8 oz. bottle.

TO USE: Rub all over your body as often as you like since this oil is an excellent skin food.

The Bath

IF YOU LIKE BATHS and want to know more about them and their history, read *The Bath Book* by Gregory and Beverly Frazier. The authors quote a bit of Antiphanes who mentions the uses of herbs in the bath:

> . . . *He really bathes*
> *In a large gilded tub, and steeps his feet*
> *And legs in rich Egyptian unguents;*
> *His jaws and breast he rubs with thick palm oil,*
> *And both his arms with extract sweet of mint;*
> *His eyebrows and his hair with marjoram,*
> *His knees and neck with essence of ground thyme* . . .

There are many kinds of baths that one can take. The addition of herbs to the bath water can make a soothing bath, a healing bath, relaxing bath, stimulating bath, a bath to improve the circulation or a toning bath. You can take an oil bath, a sand bath, a sun bath, a sea bath, a circulating bath, a mineral bath, an herb bath, a nourishing bath, a milk bath, a vinegar bath, a sauna bath, a steam bath, a sitz bath, a whirlpool bath, or an aroma bath.

My favorite bath is an herb bath of equal quantities of Comfrey, Ginseng, Mint, Lavender, Rose, and Rosemary. I soak for 30 minutes or more and rub myself with a muslin bag filled with the herbs, a cold rinse, and then I wrap up in a giant terry towel and walk about the house until dry. It's terrifically energizing.

The Body

A Simple Bath Mixture
For Stimulating the Skin

INGREDIENTS:

1 C *Peppermint leaves,* CS
1 C *Comfrey leaves,* CS
½ C *Licorice root,* CS
¼ C *Ginseng root,* PO

Variation:

1 oz. *Mint,* CS
1 oz. *Sage,* CS
1 oz. *Rosemary,* WH
1 oz. *Comfrey leaves,* CS

QUANTITY: Makes 3-5 baths.

TO MAKE: Mix all ingredients completely and store in an attractive apothecary jar in your bathroom.

TO USE: When you wish to take the stimulating bath, drop a handful of the mixed herbs into a bath ball, muslin bag or directly into the tub. Run your bath as hot as possible and step in and soak for 10-15 minutes. Then take a bristle bath brush or a Loofah and with brisk but firm circular movements, starting at the toes, rub your body from toes to nose. Always move in an upward and circular motion. Let the water run out and rinse with cool or better yet, cold water. Wrap in a towel but do not dry yourself and walk about your house or do light exercises until dry.

TIP No. 1: To stimulate your digestion or if you have had too much to drink, take a teaspoonful of these mixed herbs and place in a small prewarmed teapot. Add about 1 teaspoonful of Orange or Sage Honey. Add about 1½ cups of boiling water and steep for 5-10 minutes. Strain the tea and drink for your disordered digestion.

TIP No. 2: This herbal mixture may be reused even after having been soaked in a tub. Simply take the bag, rinse it in clear water, and store in the refrigerator. Reuse it as above within a day or two.

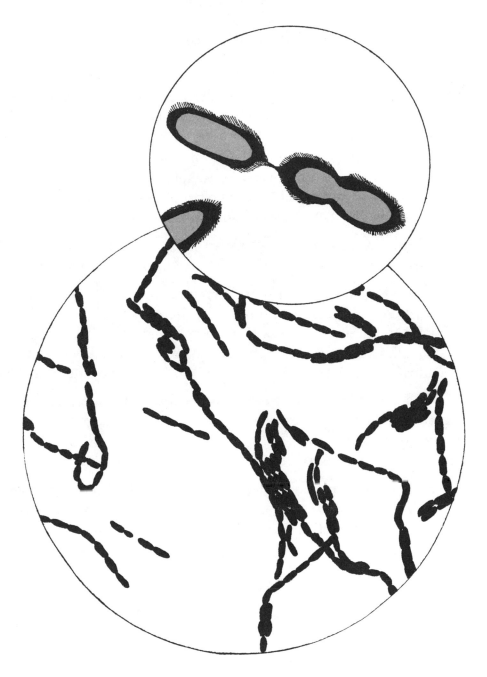

Yogurt *Lactobacillus acidophilus* detail of single bacilli (from an electron micrographic study)

Yogurt
The Fountain of Youth

WONDERFUL, HEALTHFUL YOGURT, formed by the beneficial action of certain bacteria on milk. Is it stretching a book on herbs to include Yogurt, this most fantastic of foods? Yes, of course, but then why not! Cows eat the herbage that ultimately form the milk that is worked on by the little bacteria beasties. In my household Yogurt is the first remedy that I think of for any problem, medicinal or cosmetic. It is easy to use and always available. If Yogurt is not available then we use Honey.

Yogurt can be applied directly to face and body as a cream and moisturizer. It can also be used on the eyes in case of irritation.

Yogurt should be included in everyone's daily diet to give clear skin and sparkling, youthful eyes. It is an excellent application for a burn or sunburn. Mixed with any powdered herb and applied to a clean, moist face it makes a healing, cleansing facial mask. Yogurt facials have a slight bleaching action and can, in time, even tone down unwanted freckles.

I am told that the ancient Mongols believed that certain forms of Yogurt would relax the nerves (calcium), regrow thinning hair (protein), and keep a person healthy and happy. Yogurt is not only excellent food for the complexion but will help you to get to sleep at night.

William of Rubruck in 1253 said that an intoxicating Yogurt drink called *kumiss* goes down very pleasantly, intoxicates weak brains, is very heady and powerful. This drink was also used medicinally.

Yogurt–Garlic Cleanser

INGREDIENTS:
Some *Yogurt*
1 *Garlic clove*
1 C *Water*

TO MAKE: Crush the Garlic and add it to some Yogurt. Let this steep for a few hours. Boil the water and add it to the Yogurt. Shake it around until you get a milky liquid. Strain through cheesecloth to remove all the Garlic particles.

TO USE: This liquid can be used as a cleansing, medicating vaginal douche. It will ease the itch of any sort of vaginal problem as well as helping to clear up the problem. This Yogurt-Garlic liquid can also be drunk and will act as a cleanser to the entire digestive system.

TIP: Use the Yogurt-Garlic mixture without water as an external application for sores or acne.

Yogurt–Honey Mask

INGREDIENTS:
1 T *Yogurt*
1 T *Honey*

TO MAKE: Add the two ingredients together and apply to a clean, moist face.

TO USE: Pat this mask onto the skin for a moisturizing, penetrating, hydrating, soothing application that will also help to clear up skin problems.

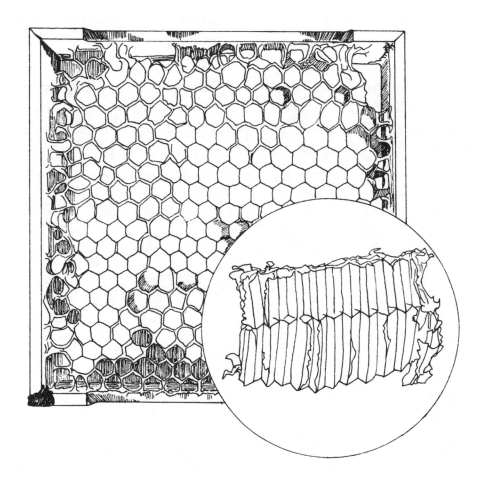

Honeycomb and Cross Section

Honey
Food for the Gods

HONEY IS A deliciously sweet substance made by Honey bees from flower nectar. Each flower or plant produces a unique Honey with a different color and flavor. Sage Honey is light and mild while Honey made from Buckwheat is stronger and darker. Most Honey sold in the United States is either Orange Honey from Orange blossoms or Clover Honey from Red Clover or White Clover plants. Honey is a perfect dressing for any and all external skin problems and is used in cosmetics as an astringent and moisturizer.

Ancient man knew the value of Honey, as food and medicine, and it appears in a carving on a wall in Valencia, Spain. The wall dates to 7000 B.C. and shows a man gathering Honey while bees fly all around him. It was used as a religious symbol. Man did not know exactly how it was produced so he worshiped Honey as a gift from the Gods and gave it mystical powers. Zeus, father of the Greek Gods was raised on Honey and goat's milk and he poured Honey from the skies to raise the dead. The Egyptians often embalmed bodies in Honey. They knew that these Honey-embalmed bodies would not decompose. And we now know that bacteria will not grow in Honey and thus it makes an excellent medium for homemade cosmetics. Hazel Berto, in *Cooking With Honey*, 1972, says:

> Thus honey held an important place in early civilizations: cleansing the spirit, heart, mind, and the body in life, and bringing the slumber of peace in death.

In our house we use Honey for its anesthetic value on little sores and wounds and use it directly on the skin as a cleansing facial mask. Apply it to athlete's foot or to acne or mix a little with your favorite lotion.

Garlicked Honey

INGREDIENTS:
Garlic cloves
Honey

TO MAKE: Peel Garlic cloves and put them in a jar. Add Honey, a little at a time over a couple of days until the jar is full. Set in a warm window for 2 weeks to a month or until the Garlic has turned somewhat opaque and all the Garlic flavor has been transferred to the Honey.

TO USE: This Garlic Honey is an excellent cough syrup. Just take a teaspoonful every couple of hours or whenever it seems necessary. You must remember though that the Honey has a lot of concentrated Garlic power in it and one teaspoonful can represent many cloves of Garlic. If you are giving this syrup to a child, you should dilute each spoonful with a bit of water. Garlic Honey also soothes a sore throat. As an application for acne or herpes it has no equal because it is both healing, soothing and slightly anesthetic. I also like to baste chicken with Garlic Honey, it's delicious.

TIP: You have to add the Honey very slowly to the jar full of Garlic because it takes time for the thick Honey to totally fill all the spaces between the Garlic cloves. Honey liquefies as it absorbs the Garlic juices and the Garlic gets rather limp and almost tasteless in time.

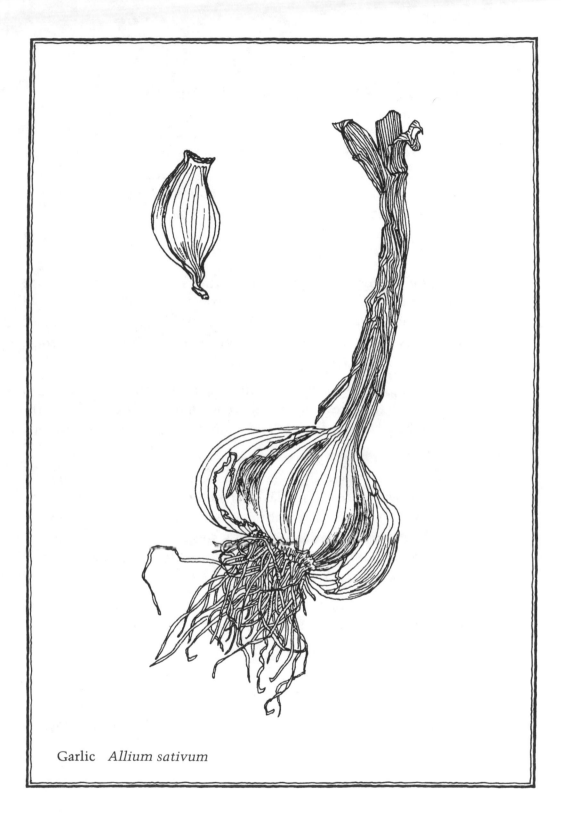

Garlic *Allium sativum*

Garlic
Great Health Restorer and Sickness Preventer

I LOVE GARLIC and I love to eat Garlic. We use it daily in the house for its known medicinal qualities.* It is most definitely a vermifuge, antiseptic, diaphoretic, diuretic, stimulant and expectorant. I have *not* used it externally as a cosmetic although it has great value when applied as a topical ointment to skin conditions such as acne or other types of pimples.

Our favorite way to use the Garlic, nature's miracle medicine, is to eat it daily in tortillas. Fry tortillas in a little corn oil, drain them, fold them, add Yogurt or mayonnaise, Alfalfa sprouts, chopped Garlic, sliced Avocado, beans if you have them and whatever else might be of interest. I probably eat 3-5 raw Garlic cloves a day.

If you have a cold, substitute Garlic soup for the traditional chicken broth. If you wish to impress a renowned chef, make Garlic chicken with a freshly butchered bird. Add salad and wine and you have a meal fit for a king. Divine!

Ancient Egyptians ate Garlic and it is said that the great tombs of the Egyptian pharaohs could not have been built but for the strength the Israelites gained from their daily ration of Garlic and Onion. Garlic was a symbol of the cosmos as manifested by its successive layers of skin that form the bulb. The Greeks and the Romans also ate of this magical herb. They used it as a health protector and aphrodisiac.

Garlic is used internally to protect a body from disease and externally as an antiseptic to protect the skin from germs and disease.

---

*Read *The Book of Garlic* by Lloyd J. Harris, (see bibliography) for a broad and detailed look at garlic in medicine, food and folklore. It is my basic reference book on the subject.

Garlic Soup
A Cosmetic that Works
from the Inside to the Outside

INGREDIENTS:

1 *Garlic bulb,* coarsely
   chopped
2 tsp. *Olive oil*
4 C good *Chicken broth*

2-4 *Egg yolks,* beaten
½ C dry *Red Wine*
   (optional)

QUANTITY: Serves 4-6.

TO MAKE: Saute the chopped Garlic in the Olive oil until translucent and tender. It is not necessary to peel the individual cloves. Add the chicken broth. Bring to a slow boil, then reduce the heat and simmer gently until the Garlic is mushy, about 30 minutes. Push through a potato ricer or strainer into a small pot. Add the beaten egg yolks slowly, stirring all the while. Return to the heat until thickened, add the wine slowly. When all is incorporated serve or chill, it is delicious either way.

TO USE: Serve the soup with dollops of Yogurt, or sour cream and chopped Almonds. It may be eaten as a main course with bread and a salad, or by itself as a health tonic.

WHY: This recipe is included for those squeamish souls who cannot eat Garlic straight. Garlic soup leaves no odor on the breath.

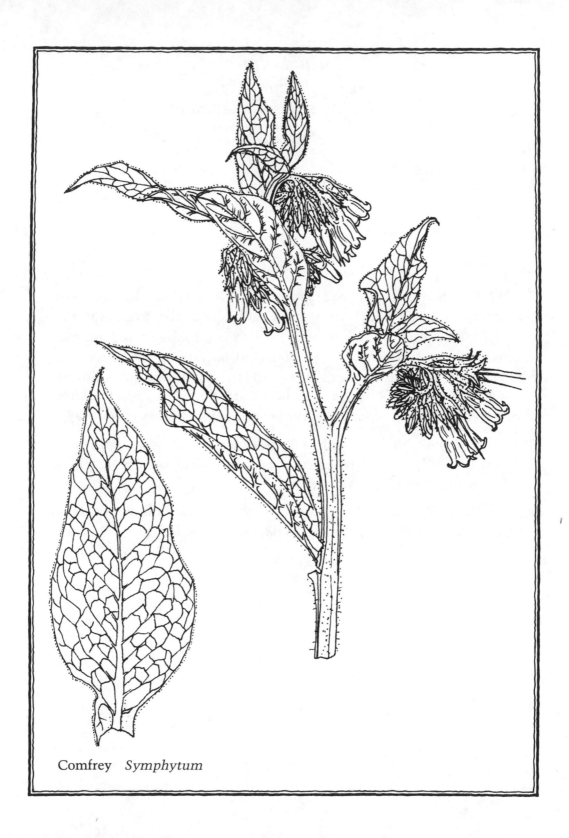

Comfrey *Symphytum*

Comfrey

COMFREY IS A great healer. It has great powers to heal the body internally and externally. Medical doctors use this plant in the form of an extract from the leaf and root called allantoin. *A Consumer's Dictionary of Cosmetic Ingredients* says:

> Allantoin: Used in cold creams, hand lotions, hair lotions, after-shave lotions, and other skin-soothing cosmetics because of its ability to help heal wounds and skin ulcers and to stimulate the growth of healthy tissue. Colorless crystals, soluble in hot water, it is prepared synthetically by the oxidation of uric acid . . . or by heating uric acid with dichloroacetic acid. It is non toxic.

Herbalists do not have to resort to the use of synthetic allantoin. We can get Comfrey for a few dollars a pound at the local herb store. We use either the leaf or the root in cut or powdered form. The powdered root is taken internally in capsules, the cut root is decocted and drunk, or applied externally. The leaf infusion is taken for ulcers, blood circulation or arthritis and added to all cosmetic herbal mixtures for its wonderfully healing, soothing and astringent effect. Here again we have an herb that has a twofold use, it is both a soothing healer *and* an astringent. Perfect for all types of complexions from dry to oily. We use it in facial steam herbs, and all lotions and creams, bath mixtures, shampoos, facial masks or topical applications.

Use it medicinally as a cell-regenerative to deal with any wound, abscess, ulcer, burn, in everything and anything that you can think of. You can't go wrong using Comfrey.

An Herbal Shower Bath for Lower Back Ache

INGREDIENTS:

1 C *Rosemary leaves*

1 C *Sage leaves*

1 C *Strawberry leaves*

1 C *Comfrey root, CS*

1 C *Comfrey leaves*

1 C *Lavender buds*

QUANTITY: Makes 4-6 baths or showers.

TO MAKE: Use only dried herbs, mix them together and place in some sort of container for future use.

TO USE: Take a generous handful of herbs and place in a muslin bag. Soak the bag in a small amount of water until the herbs are completely wet. Start your shower warm, gradually working up to hot, and then place the spray on 'needle'. Alternate 'needling' your lower back and bottom for 1 minute on hot, then turn to cold for 20 seconds. While doing this, rub your body with the herb-filled bag in circular motions from the toes up, concentrating on the aching area. Complete your shower by taking a 30-second cold rinse, as cold as comfortably possible. Wipe yourself all over with the herb-filled bag.

WHY: This mixture of herbs and the technique of hot and cold showers opens the pores, stimulates the body's circulation, thereby ridding it of accumulated toxins.

TIP: In summer, if you are growing your own herbs, substitute the fresh and aromatic herbs for the dried ones. Of course, you should make only enough for 1 shower as fresh herbs will not keep for more than a day once moistened. Pick a small bit of each of the herbs, place in your muslin bag and scrub away at your body, as in the above directions.

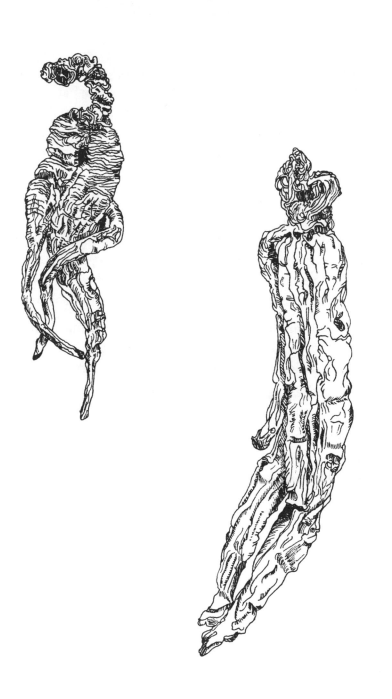

Ginseng *Panax quinquefolium*

Ginseng

AFTER HEARING ABOUT the wonder of Ginseng* as a tonic, I decided that as an experiment I would try it for awhile and see what would happen. So during a three month period about three years ago, I took a daily dose of ⅛ to ¼ oz. of the root in capsule form. I can't say that I felt any better. Actually, I like the combination of good food, vitamins, exercise and a bit of garlic for my daily routine.

Asiatic Ginseng has been known and used for over 6000 years. It has been called the manroot, five fingers, oriental panacea and other common names. The plant itself is a rather rare perennial that sets seeds which take 18 months to germinate. In about six years, the plant is 8-10 inches high with 2-4 leaves each divided into five leaflets. The flowers are quite small and the roots large and nicely aromatic. It grows in cool and damp woods.

Much study and experiment has determined that Ginseng definitely acts as a tonic and stimulant. It has also been used as an aphrodisiac, for birth control, colds, headaches, fevers, poor circulation, vomiting, arthritis, rheumatism, as a blood coagulant and for respiratory problems.

Ginseng has been shown to be nontoxic even in large doses, increases a person's resistance to a wide variety of physical and biological stresses, is a normalizer and improves a person's physical and mental efficiency. This alone should make you want to add Ginseng to your daily diet.

---

*For more information, read the following Ginseng books: *The Book of Ginseng* by Sarah Harriman or *The Ginseng Book* by Louise Veninga.

Ginseng Tonic Tea

INGREDIENTS:
½ oz. *Ginseng root*
1 T *Honey*
2 C *Water*

TO MAKE: Bring all the ingredients to a boil and simmer for 5-10 minutes. Remove from heat and cool until drinkable. Drink 1 cup warm in the morning and the other cup cold at night.

TO USE: Drink this tea when in a period of stress and continue its use for no more than 10 days. The Ginseng itself can be reboiled several times although the more you boil it the less pleasant the taste. But at Ginseng prices, you can probably stand the taste.

Ginseng Bath Herb Mixture

INGREDIENTS:
½ oz. *Ginseng*, PO
1 oz. *Rose petals*, WH
1 oz. *Comfrey root*
   or *leaf*, CS

1 oz. *Almond meal*
1 oz. *Orange peel*, CS
1 oz. *Red Clover*, CS

QUANTITY: Use about ½ oz. per bath. Makes 8-12 baths.

TO MAKE: Mix all the ingredients together and store away.

TO USE: Follow any of the bath directions such as those on p. 85.

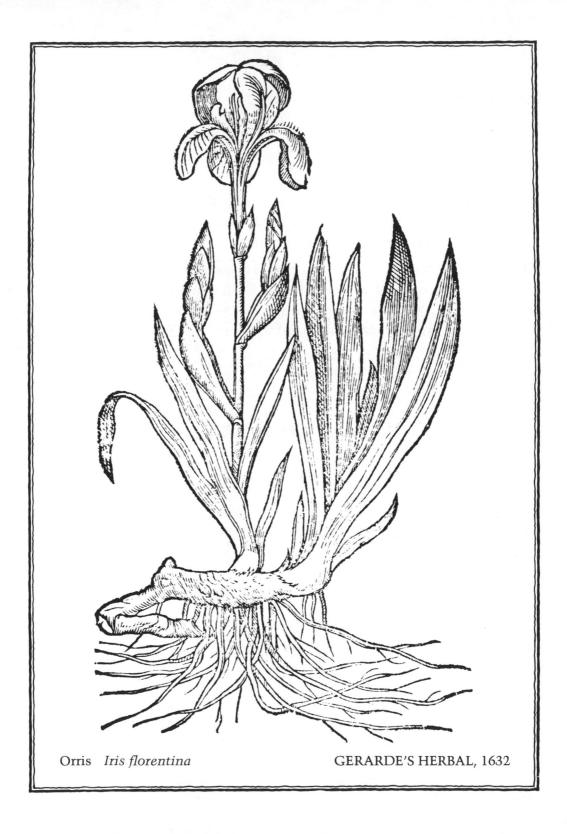

Orris   *Iris florentina*   GERARDE'S HERBAL, 1632

Orris

The Fragrant Rhizomes of Iris germanica, I. florentina *and* I. pallida

This iris is planted, allowed to mature, and then is removed from the ground and the rhizome, called Orris root, is broken up. Some of the rhizome is replanted to restock the bed. The rest is allowed to dry completely and rest for as long as two years during which time the violet scent develops. The scent often intensifies even after this time. Over a year ago when I moved and enlarged my Orris bed, I dried a few small pieces. I was rather surprised when it seemed that there would be no scent. However, having just now broken open a piece of the rhizome it indeed smells divine.

This rhizome has extensive use as a fixative in perfumery. The scent develops with time and is useful in potpourris and sachets. It makes an excellent body or deodorant powder although some folks have an allergic reaction to its use. Orris is also used in the bath, toothpowders, in creams, lotions, hand care products and hair care products.

Orris Dry Shampoo

Mix together equal quantities of Orris powder and cornmeal. Part your hair in sections and sprinkle this absorbent powder onto the scalp. Bend over at the waist and stroke and massage the scalp with the fingers; with a bristle brush, brush all the powder out. Your hair and scalp will be clean and fragrant.

Cleo's Bath Milk

INGREDIENTS:
1 C non-fat *Milk*
½ C *Almond meal*
½ C *Orris root*, PO

TO MAKE: Put all the above ingredients into a blender and blend on low until it is completely incorporated. Or beat with a wire whisk or egg beater.

TO USE: Run a warm bath and pour the Bath Milk into the tub. Soak and relax. Take the opportunity to rest your eyes with herbal pads. Wash as usual.

A Perfumed Body Powder

Take Orange Flowers, a pound; common Roses picked without the Yellow Pedicles, a pound; Clove July-flowers picked with the White End of their Leaves cut off, half a pound: Marjoram, and Myrtle Leaves picked, of each half a pound; Musk Roses, Thyme, Lavender, Rosemary, Sage, Chamomile, Melilot, Hyssop, Sweet Basil, and Balm of each two ounces; fifteen or twenty Bay Leaves, two or three handfuls of Jasmin, as many little Green Oranges, and half a pound of Salt. Put them in a proper vessel, and leave them together a whole month, carefully observing to stir the mixture well twice a day with a wooden spatula or spoon.

At the month's end, add twelve ounces of Florentine Orris-root in fine powder, and the same quantity of powdered Benzoin, of Cloves, and Cinnamon finely powdered, each two ounces; Mace, Storax, Calamus Aromaticus, all in fine powder, and Cypress-powder, of each an ounce; Yellow Sanders and Cyprus or Sweet Flag, of each three-quarters ounce.

–*From* The Toilet of Flora, *1779*

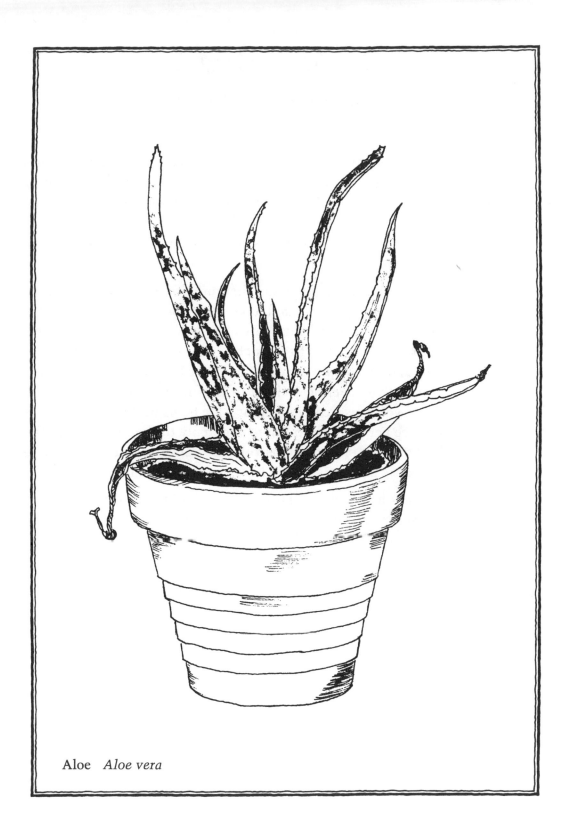

Aloe   *Aloe vera*

Aloe Vera

An Ancient Wonder Plant

ALOE VERA, or true Aloe. Mentioned in the Bible, drawn on Egyptian tombs, brought to the New World by the Spaniards and used by country doctors and present-day herbalists, the Aloe has been used in much the same manner for centuries. It is a remedy for insect bites, rashes, swellings, ringworm, peptic ulcer, burns, boils, blisters, body odor, cuts, scratches or sunburn.

It has great value in the home as a first rate first-aid remedy for burns or scalds. If you have your own plant, take a large basal leaf and peel away the outer green rind to reveal the shiny clear gel. Apply this gel directly to the sore or burn. Or cut off two inches of leaf and slice it in half to reveal the gel and then apply the cut side to the hurt area. The Aloe will provide a protective covering and aid in the immediate healing of the area. However, you must remember that Aloe helps heal fast, so fast that the area must be perfectly clean before you apply the gel. Do not use the greenish brown juice of the rind as this substance containing Aloin is used as a cathartic and can severely irritate a wound or burn.

If you do not have your own plant, Aloe is sold in health food stores and herb shops in the form of juice or gel. (Aloe Vera Gel is distributed by Aloe Products, Inc., P.O. Box 424, Hunt, Texas 78024.)

If you can get a plant, plop it in some succulent soil, water it once a week and soon the plant will become adjusted to its new home and develop new roots. Even if brown and dry, wait, don't overwater, and it will become a nice large house plant.

Old-Fashioned Cold Cream with Aloe Vera

INGREDIENTS:

1 oz. *Lanolin,* liquid
   measure

3 oz. *Almond oil*

2 oz. *Rosewater*

2 T or more *Aloe gel*

QUANTITY: Makes a 2 month's supply of cream when used daily.

TO MAKE: In a blender or with a beater thoroughly incorporate the Aloe gel and the Almond oil, and pour into a small enamel pot. Using a double boiler or water bath, melt it together with the lanolin. Remove from the heat and add the Rosewater, beating continuously until the mixture has cooled. Pour or spoon into a cream jar.

TO USE: Apply this cream as body cream, healing application for pimples or simply as a night-time moisturizer.

TIP: If you do not have a double boiler, one can be fashioned easily enough with materials that you might have at hand. Take a small enamel pot and set it in a larger pot that contains water. Put both of these over the heat and *voila,* you have an old-fashioned double boiler, also called a water bath or *bain marie.*

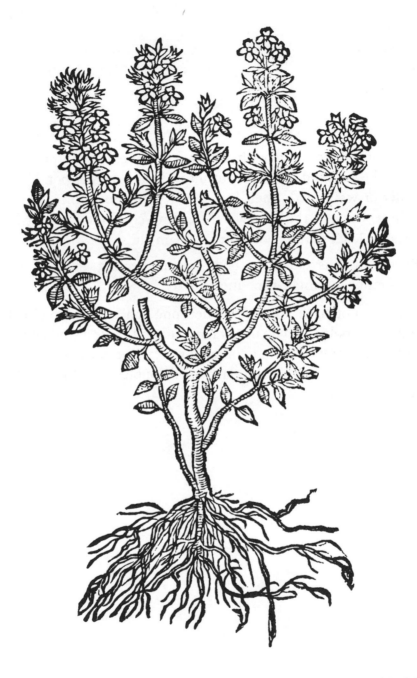

Thyme   *Thymus vulgaris*   GERARDE'S HERBAL, 1632

Thyme

THYMES ARE SMALL, bushy plants, pungently aromatic, with small leaves that exude the scent. Depending on the species or variety of Thyme, the scent can range from the typical culinary Thyme to Lemon, Camphor, Turpentine, Caraway, Nutmeg, Licorice or Mint. There are sixty or so varieties of Thyme, each with its own particular scent and flavor. I am particularly fond of the small and dainty *Thymus Herba-barona*, the Caraway Thyme, and grow it along the ground near my Caraway plant.

The little Thymes like deep rich soil as they use much of the earth's nourishment. Grow it near your cabbages or *Brassicas* in the garden as a companion plant to repel the cabbage moth. Grow *Thymus vulgaris* as a border plant to attract bees. Thyme Honey is very rich, thick and dark and excellent when mixed with water as an antiseptic cough syrup.

Some Basic Thyme Recipes

Add 1 cup of Thyme leaves to your bath—it is strengthening to the body. Mix it with an equal quantity of Lavender and Comfrey and use ½ cup of this mixture to steam the face, to rinse the hair, or as a fragrant, astringent douche.

Medicinally, Thyme is a warming herb and is used for colds, coughs, respiratory ailments, for cramps and colic, as a tonic, antiseptic, slight anesthetic, as a spray to deodorize, or for skin diseases such as exzema. *Thymol* (from Thyme oil) is a powerful antiseptic and deodorant. Thyme oil is often used in perfumery as it is cheap and the scent goes a long way. It is mainly used for soaps.

A fine mixture of herbs for the bath or to steam the face is: Camomile to reduce puffiness, Licorice to relax the pores and open them for cleaning, Comfrey as a cellular regenerative, and Thyme as an antiseptic.

Foot Balm

INGREDIENTS:

¼ C thick infusion of
 Marigold

¼ C thick infusion
 of *Thyme*

¼ C anhydrous *Lanolin*

¼ C *Listerine*

TO MAKE: Make your infusions (see p. 17), strain them, add them to a pot containing the lanolin. Set the pot in a water bath and heat and beat until the lanolin melts. Remove pots from the heat, remove pot from the water bath, add the listerine and beat with a small wooden spoon until cool. Pour or spoon into cream jar, cover and shake until cold.

TO USE: After your bath or shower, shake excess water from the feet and rub the Foot Balm onto the moist feet.

WHY: This mixture is cooling and healing to tired, achy feet.

Help For Athlete's Foot

Athlete's foot is an itchy fungus infection that can generally be cured by correcting the acid balance of the skin in the toe area. The fungus will only thrive in a moist, dark, alkaline environment and if you change this environment then you can usually cure the disease. You must keep your feet clean and DRY. Wash them twice a day with an acid-balanced soap and dry them thoroughly. Powder them with Orris root. In the morning give them a vinegar and water soak, 1 T apple cider vinegar to 1 cup of warm water. In the evening soak them in a warm thick infusion of Red Clover, Thyme and Violets for 20 minutes. Give them sun, light and air. Keep your shoes dry and powdered. Wear only white cotton socks that have been boiled before wearing.

Simple Massage Oil for Aching Legs and Feet

INGREDIENTS:
1 quart of mixed *Oils*
¼ oz. *oil of Sage* (approx. 1 tsp.)
¼ oz. *oil of Rosemary* (approx. 1 tsp.)

TO MAKE: Pour the essential oils into the mixed vegetable oils, shake thoroughly and set aside for a few days while the scent develops.

TO USE: Take a bit of the Massage Oil into your palm and warm it by rubbing your hands together gently. Then massage into the feet and legs by rubbing, squeezing, pounding and kneading with the hands. Rub the oil up, down and around each toe, knead into the arch, and press into heel; squeeze around the achilles tendon and then massage up onto the leg and calf with large swirling motions. Take at least 5 minutes or more for each foot and leg. Your feet will feel ever so much better for the massage and quite revived from the attention they have received.

TIP: If the oil seems too strongly scented for you, increase the amount of vegetable oil to 5 cups or decrease the essential oils to 1 teaspoon per quart.

P.S.   This oil is terrific for aching tired muscles anywhere on the body, or for dry flaky skin on the legs.

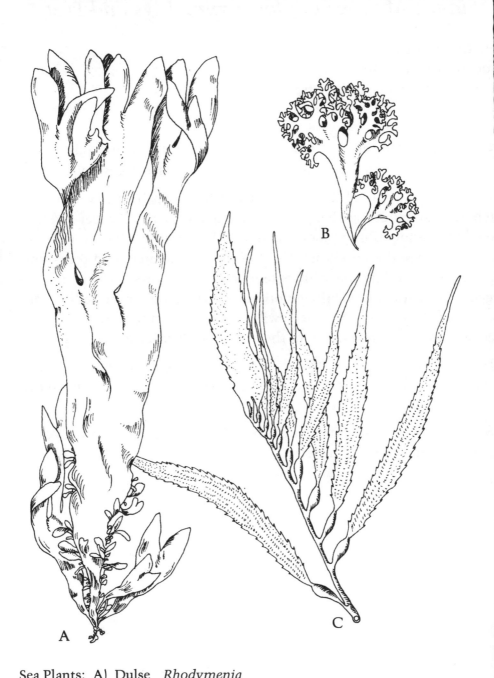

Sea Plants: A) Dulse *Rhodymenia*
B) Irish Moss *Chrondrus crispus*
C) Kelp *Macrocytis integrifolia*

Sea Plants

Sᴇᴀ ᴘʟᴀɴᴛꜱ ᴀʀᴇ commonly known by the names Algae, Seaweed, or Kelp. All kelps are seaweed but not all seaweeds are kelp. Sea plants are richer in calcium than land plants and very high in potassium. Sea plants contain all the nutrients needed by man and are a healthful addition to the diet. When you go to your local herb store you will find that in general only three sea plants are available. These three we will discuss briefly.

DULSE: Dulse belongs to a large group called the red algae. This group also includes Irish Moss and some red algae that contain extracts called *agar agar.* Dulse is the sea plant most often eaten. It is tender, red, and goes well in salads or shredded and sprinkled on vegetables. Dulse is used in teas and other herbal mixtures to supply the essential micro-nutrients. It is especially useful in teas for those who are fasting or dieting.

IRISH MOSS: This type is a member of the red algae as is Dulse. It is used as a demulcent, emollient, and nutritive. Boiled with water it forms a jelly that is a useful base for creams, lotions or toothpaste. It, as well as other red algae, furnishes the extract Carrageenen used in commercial desserts, and as a stabilizer and emulsifier in cosmetics and creams.

KELP: Kelp is a name given to the large group of the brown algae. This includes *Laminaria, Macrocystis, Nereocystis,* the bladder Kelp and *Fucus.* The Kelp are generally used externally in cosmetics, as poultices, or powdered and added to mineral baths. They are used in lotions and creams for skin disease, and to make sea-pod liniment which is used for massage to diminish fat and remove what some people call cellulite, as in saddlebag thighs.

Seaweed Leg Gel

INGREDIENTS:

1 tsp. *Irish Moss*
1 C *Herbal Infusion* made with
    Lemon, Witch Hazel and
    Comfrey
2 oz. *Bay Rum* or *Listerine* (al-
    cohol)

TO MAKE: Make the Herbal Infusion, strain the liquid and add it to the Irish Moss in a small pot. Simmer with a closed lid for 20 minutes or until the moss is soft, gooey and jelly-like. Strain through cheesecloth. Add the alcohol as a preservative. Mix together.

TO USE: Massage into the legs with upward strokes. Very refreshing and especially suitable for those who sit a great deal.

TIP: Don't forget to check this book for other sea plant recipes. I use them in herbal steam facials to provide an external source of necessary micro-nutrients. I also use them in homemade toothpaste (see page 61).

Sea Salt Bath

INGREDIENTS:

Mix equal quantities of *Salt,* pow-
    dered *Dulse, Baking Soda*
    and *Epsom Salts.*

TO USE: Pour a goodly quantity (at least 1 cup) in a warm bath. Soak and let the healing salts release the toxins and poisons from your skin. This bath is very relaxing and soothing.

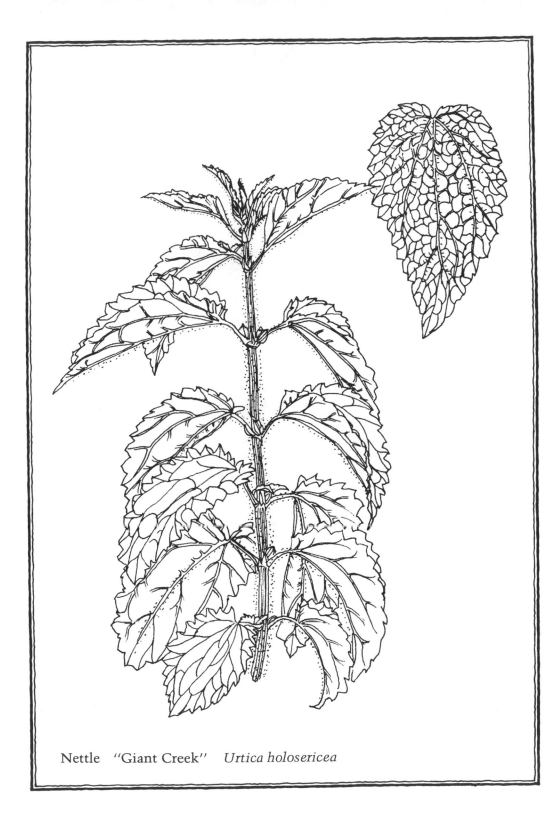

Nettle   "Giant Creek"   *Urtica holosericea*

Nettle

A ROMAN HISTORIAN said this of the Nettle:

> The soldiers brought some of the nettle seed with them and sowed it there for their use to rub and chaff their limbs, when through extreme cold they should be stiff or benumbed, having been told that the climate of Britain was so cold that it was not to be endured.

These Roman soldiers serving under Julius Caesar brought the nettle from their native land as a stimulant for the circulation and a specific remedy for the legs.

Nettle generally grows to about 3 feet but in compatible situations will grow as tall as 8 feet. It flowers in the summer and here in California covers many hills.

It can be eaten as it is rich in calcium, iron and Vitamins A and C. Nettle branches have been used as a switch to beat arthritic limbs. It has been used in the cure of bladder difficulties, anemia, kidney and liver problems, overweight, for childbirth, and as a muscle relaxant.

Cosmetically the nettle is used to stimulate hair growth, to give shine and body to the hair or as a stimulant in facial steams.

Nettle was used by the American Indians as a fabric and as twine and in other countries to make paper.

Nettle fed to animals encourages milk production or egg production. A vegetable fertilizer can be made that is most encouraging to the growth of house plants.

House Plant Fertilizer

INGREDIENTS:
1 oz. *Nettle*
1 oz. *Comfrey root*
1 oz. *Kelp*

TO MAKE: Put the herbs in a gallon jug and fill it with water. Steep for at least a day before using. Pour the water from the jug onto the plants instead of their regular watering. Add more water to the jug as it is emptied. You may refill the jug for as long as 10 days. Then use the herbs themselves as compost or mulch.

Herb Bath
Especially for Poor Circulation in the Legs

INGREDIENTS:

1 oz. *Nettle leaves,*
   dried
1 oz. *Kelp*

1 oz. *Comfrey root*
   or *leaf*
1 oz. *Lavender*

QUANTITY: 3 to 4 baths.

TO MAKE: Mix all these dried herbs and store them away for use.

TO USE: To really stimulate the circulation, first rub your body all over with a rough towel or a Loofah. In the meantime put a handful of the mixed herbs into a muslin bag and drop into the tub. Run a warm to hot bath and get in. Rub your body with the muslin bag, up from the toes and down from the nose. Stay in the bath about 30 minutes. Take a cold shower. Rub yourself dry with a rough Turkish towel. Rest on a slant-board.

Where To Buy It
Drop In or Write for a Catalog and Mail-order

CALIFORNIA

Greentree Grocers—3560 Mt. Acadia Blvd. San Diego, CA 92111. A wonderful store with lots of amenities. Ask Julia about good books for living the healthy life.

Herb Products Co.—11012 Magnolia Blvd. No. Hollywood, CA 91601. Everything you need to make all your own fabulous herbal body-care products. $1.00 for catalog.

Herbal BodyWorks/Herbal Studies Course by Correspondence—219 Carl Street. San Francisco, CA 94117. A good resource for all your herbal questions. Send $3.00 and a SASE* and your question regarding where to get whatever it is you want. "All Things Herbal" are the questions answered. Send $1.00 for the correspondance course information.

Herbal Effect—616 Lighthouse Ave. Monterey, CA 93940. A wonderful store and a fabulous mail-order catalog for all your herbal needs. $1.00 for catalog.

San Francisco Herb & Natural Food/Nature's Herb Company—1010 46th St. Emeryville CA 94608. A good mail-order catalog for everything about herbs. $1.00

INDIANA

Greenfield Herb Garden—P.O. Box 437. Shipshewana, IN 46565. Catalog available.

IOWA

Frontier Cooperative Herbs—A wonderful mail-order catalog that is free to all who request it. Not a terrific selection of books but everything else herbal is well represented. Good quality, reasonably priced essential oils.

NEW YORK

Enchantments, Inc.—341 East 9th Street. New York, NY 10003. Many, many interesting items that include all necessary ingredients for your special home-made body-care products. $2.00 for mail-order catalog.

OHIO

WoodSpirits Herb Shop—1920 Apple Rd. St. Paris, OH 43072. Fabulous hand-milled soap. Barbara also teaches classes in the healthful uses of herbs. Mail-order catalog $1.00

*Self-Addressed Stamped Envelope

OREGON

Goodwin Creek's Secret Garden— P.O. Box 83. Williams, OR 97544. Wonderful plants and seeds and a collection of products and books. Mail-order catalog $1.00.

TEXAS

Varney's Chemist Laden—310 East Main Street. Fredericksburg, TX 78624. Wonderful products in a beautiful store. Classes and a delicious Herbal Bed & Breakfast Inn. Mail-order catalog $1.00

VERMONT

Rathdowney, Ltd.—P.O. Box 357. Bethel, VT 05032. This is a full-service herb shop and apothecary. Lots of unique products and books that might be difficult to find elsewhere. The display gardens are at 3 River Street in Bethel. No charge for the catalog.

WASHINGTON

The HerbFarm—32804 Issaquah-Fall City Road. Fall City, WA 98024. Products, classes, books, ingredients. A lovely mail-order catalog with many products you will not find elsewhere.

WISCONSIN

The Soap Opera—312 State St. Madison, WI 53703. Great stuff and an excellent assortment of herbal massage oils.

OUT OF COUNTRY

AUSTRALIA

The Fragrant Garden—Portsmouth Rd. Erina, NSW 2250. $2.00 for mail-order catalog.

CANADA

True Essence Aromatherapy Ltd.—1910 Bowness Road NW. Calgary, Alberta, T2N3K6. No charge for the wonderful mail-order catalog. Wow! They have everything. This company is run by a truly ethical person.

ENGLAND

Culpeper The Herbalist—Hadstock Road, Linson, Cambridge CB16NJ. $1.00 for a fabulous mail-order catalog of everything natural.

A Glossary of Cosmetic Terms

Alcohol. Used in many cosmetics as an antiseptic astringent. Cools the skin as it evaporates. Very drying and not recommended.

Astringent. Any substance that tightens the pores of the skin, such as alcohol. An astringent does not have to be painful but can be soothing, such as Rosewater or Almond meal. Astringents are generally used on oily skin but herbal astringents can be used by everyone.

Baking Soda. A water-soluble white crystalline substance available in any supermarket and used in baths for itchy skin, as a soothing soak for irritated skin conditions, or as simple tooth powder.

Barley. A grass used in baths to soothe and soften skin.

Beeswax. A substance secreted by bees to build the walls of their cells and used by cosmetic manufacturers as an emulsifier to soften and protect skin. It is said *not* to clog the pores.

Benzoin. A resin from trees, used as a natural preservative in cosmetics and a fixative in perfumes and potpourris.

Borax. A water softener, preservative and natural texturizer in creams for the body or cold creams. Used in cosmetics as an emulsifier and diluted, it is used to soothe irritated skin. Has an alkaline pH.

Boric Acid. An antiseptic, bactericide and fungicide *not* to be used on babies or ingested or inhaled by anyone.

Camphor. A crystalline substance obtained from the camphor tree used as an antiseptic and counter-irritant. If inhaled for too long a time it can give you a fierce headache.

Castile Soap. A soap made from at least 40% olive oil.

Castor Oil. An oil from the castor bean used in many cosmetics. It is an emollient that forms a hard film when dry, and is often used in lipsticks.

Cerate. An ointment or cream made with oil and wax to harden it.

Cocoa Butter. A solid fat used to soften and lubricate the skin and often used in place of wax to harden creams.

Coconut Oil. A white saturated fat obtained from coconut that melts at body temperature and is used to lubricate and smoothe the skin.

Cornstarch. A starch obtained from corn kernels used as a powder for irritated skin, slick but slightly abrasive.

Diaphoretic. A substance that produces or increases perspiration.

Decoction. A mixture of herbs and water that is boiled and used internally or externally, medicinally or cosmetically.

Demulcent. A substance used internally that soothes irritated mucous membranes.

Emollient. A substance, usually slick, thick, slimy or creamy, used externally to soothe or soften the skin. Usually made from oils, water, and wax; there are also many potent emollients among the herbs.

Emulsifier. A substance that binds two dissimilar substances together such as when an egg is used with oil and vinegar to make mayonnaise.

Epsom Salts. Crystals of magnesium sulfate used in baths to "draw" toxic substances from the body through the skin. Also very effective for sore, tired muscles.

Essential Oil. In the pure sense this term means the oil that is extracted from real flowers and herbs, but the word is often used loosely to mean any perfumed oil that imitates a real scent.

Extracts. A concentrated form of any substance.

Gel. A jelly-like material like Jello, ie. the clear crystalline innards of an Aloe leaf.

Gelatin. A protein usually extracted from hooves, bones and tendons, used in cosmetics because it sticks to hair or skin.

Glycerine. Occurring naturally in soap manufacture as an emollient and humectant. Most commercial glycerine is made as by-product of the petroleum industry.

Honey. A deliciously sweet substance made by honey bees from flower nectar. Each flower or plant produces a unique honey with a different color and flavor. Honey from Sage plants is mild while honey from Buckwheat is stronger and darker. Most honey sold in the United States is either Orange Honey from Orange blossoms or Clover Honey from Red Clover plants. Honey is a perfect dressing for any and all external skin problems and is used in cosmetics as an astringent and moisturizer.

Humectant. A substance that preserves the moisture or water content of the skin. Most dry skin is lacking in moisture rather than oil and therefore humectants and moisturizers are needed rather than creams or oils. Natural glycerin and pure rosewater is one of the most effective humectants.

Infusion. A mixture of herbs and water that is soaked or steeped for a period of time and used internally or externally, medicinally or cosmetically.

Lanolin. A fat-like substance obtained from the wool of sheep that is a natural emulsifier and used in cosmetics to prevent or relieve excess dryness of the skin.

Mellite. A decoction or an infusion that you use cosmetically; it has honey added for its cosmetic effect. Also made directly from honey and herbs.

Menthol. A mild local anesthetic obtained naturally from the herb peppermint but now is mostly made synthetically.

Moisturizer. A substance that is used to add water or moisture to the skin.

Ointment. A greasy or creamy salve applied externally to the skin. It can contain herbs or other active substances for specific cosmetic or medicinal purpose.

Orange Water. When Orange blossoms and water are simmered together, the steam distillate condenses to form Orange water useful in cosmetics for dry skin.

pH. A symbol for a scale (0-14) that measures the acidity or alkalinity of a substance, ie. vinegar (a pH of 2.3) and honey, skin and hair are acid, while most soaps (8-10) and mineral waters are alkaline. Plain water and blood are either neutral (7), or very close to neutral.

Poultice. A soft, moist compress applied to a sore or inflamed part of the body.

Rosewater. The steam distillate that condenses after Roses and water are simmered together. Another way to obtain Rosewater is simply to infuse pure oil of Roses in distilled water for a number of days. When the water takes on the scent of oil, strain out the oil.

Styptic. A substance used to stop bleeding. A liquid brewed from the tea plant; or from any other herbs.

Tincture of Benzoin. An alcoholic solution of Benzoin.

Tisane. An infusion of herbs.

Zinc Oxide. Usually found as a white and creamy ointment that is used as an astringent, antiseptic and for many types of skin diseases to protect the skin.

A Selected Bibliography

Basic Guide to Formulations of Cosmetics and Toiletries. Rita Corporation. Chicago, Illinois. 1971.

Bragg, Patricia. *The Amazing New Hollywood Plan.* Health Science. Burbank, California. 1971.

Buchman, Dian Dincin. *Feed Your Face.* Duckworth & Co. Ltd., London. 1973.

Bryan, John E. & Coralie Castle. *The Edible Ornamental Garden.* 101 Productions. San Francisco, California. 1974.

Clark, Linda. *Secrets of Health and Beauty.* Pyramid Books. New York, New York. 1970.

Culpeper House. Price List. London. 1963.

de Gingins-Lassaraz, Baron Fred. *Natural History of the Lavenders.* Herb Society of America. Boston, Massachusetts. 1967.

Dussauce, Professor H. *A General Treatise on the Manufacture of Soap.* Henry Carey Baird. London. 1869.

Frazier, Gregory and Beverly. *The Bath Book.* Troubadour Press. San Francisco, California. 1973.

Harris, Lloyd J. *The Book of Garlic.* Panjandrum/Aris Books. San Francisco, California. 1975.

Heffern, Richard. *The Herb Buyer's Guide.* Pyramid Books. New York, New York. 1973.

Hewitt, James. *Facial Isometrics for Youth and Beauty in 3 Minutes Each Day.* Award Books. New York. 1970.

Homola, D.C., Samuel. *Backache: Home Treatment and Prevention.* Parker Publishing Co. West Nyack, New York. 1970.

Keller, Jeanne. *Healing with Water: Special Applications and Uses of Water in Home Remedies for Everyday Ailments.* Parker Publishing Co. West Nyack, New York. 1968.

Kneipp, Sebastian. *My Water-Cure.* Jos. Koesel. Bavaria. 1897.

Lawson, Donna. *Mother Nature's Beauty Cupboard.* Thomas Y. Crowell Company. New York. 1973.

Leyel, Mrs. C. F. *Herbal Delights.* Faber and Faber Limited. London. 1937.

The Magic of Herbs: A Modern Book of Secrets. Harcourt, Brace & Company. 1926.

Rose, Jeanne. *Herbs & Things.* Grosset & Dunlap. 1972.

The Herbal Body Book. Grosset & Dunlap. 1976.

The Modern Herbal, Putnam Publishing, New York, 1987.

The Herbal Guide to Food. North Atlantic Books, Berkeley, CA. 1989.

Index

(**Boldface** page numbers indicate the principle reference in the text)

Red Clover, **37,** 38, 41, 44, 62, 101, 110
Rinses, conditioning vinegar for face, 65;
for dandruff, 44; herbal conditioning
vinegar for light hair, 32; herbal for all
hair types, 41
Rose, **53,** 54, 55, 58, 62, 65, 66, 101, 107
Rosemary, **27,** 35, 38, 41, 44, 65, 86, 98,
111

Sage, 41, **57,** 65, 70, 86, 98, 111
Salad Dressings, 32, 65
Sea Plants, 38, 62, 63, **113,** 114, 117
Shampoos, dry, 103, herbal castile for
light hair, 29; protein herbal for dark
hair, 28
Skin, acne treatments, 91, 92, 107; healing creams 59, 107; oils, 84, 111;
steam treatment for oiliness, large

pores, dryness, itching, 60; soothing
bath mix, 114; stimulating bath mix,
86; remedy for burns, 59, 109
Strawberry, 62, **64,** 65, 98

Teas, detoxifying, 47; ginseng tonic for
stress, 101; to improve hair health, 38;
stimulating, 60, 86
Throat, cough syrup, 92; moisturizing
cream, 55; sore throat cure, 58
Thyme, **109,** 110
Toothpaste, 61

Violet, **43,** 44, 110

Witch Hazel, **40,** 41, 44, 114
Witchcraft, 40
Yogurt, **88,** 89

Notes